Personal Health Records for Governments:

2025

Federica Andreoni
and
Mohammad Al-Ubaydli

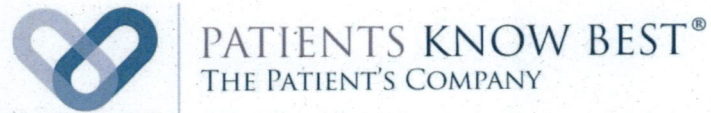

ISBN: 978-1-0686943-0-1

To government employees,
who serve their citizens quietly
even while receiving criticism loudly.

CONTENTS

FOREWORD

Digital service provision has been the primary way of reaching out to clients by the private sector for at least 20 years, even longer in some sectors and some countries. In Estonia, online banking was launched 30 years ago in 1994. By the turn of the century, visiting offices was the exception, not the norm, when subscribing to telecommunication and other well-standardised services. Estonia's online tax board was launched in 1997. Almost no one under the age of 50 has seen a taxman in Estonia.

Of course, in most countries, the digital services of the public sector had to compete initially with the traditional, appointment-based service model. Partially, this was because the digital services were not offered universally, nor linked to a single government portal, and weren't accessible with a universal digital ID. Instead, the variety of methods for access and identify verification created confusion and delayed development.

Consolidation followed in most countries. As people mostly transact online in their everyday lives, governments have had to follow the trend. So, it was no longer possible to force physical appointment-based services. While most governments still do not provide single-access universal service portals for all public service delivery, they have made sectoral advances. For example, a single digital space for business management, then social service provision, and finally, healthcare.

Citizens' control over who can see information about their health is crucial. It is less of a problem in Europe, where governments often take full responsibility for organising healthcare. The cost of insurance, therefore, does not depend on the health patterns of any individual. Instead, it is based on solidarity. In systems where all or part of the insurance cost is carried by citizens directly, there is always the risk of health profile-based prices or, in the case of high-risk patients, a lack of providers willing to deliver the service. It is hard to regulate against these risks, even if most governments try to do so.

Even in solidarity-based health insurance models, people are generally worried about who can see the sensitive data.

On the other hand, people understand that centralized healthcare databases reduce the need for different healthcare providers to perform repetitive actions. This saves time for citizens and money for the government. Therefore, it is the job of the government to provide necessary safety clauses for citizens, allowing them control over their personal health data.

For example, Estonians can donate their DNA samples to the Estonian Genome Bank in exchange for their genetic risk profile. People are free to choose whether or not to share that data with their family practitioner. For the rest of health data, citizens can verify that only their relevant healthcare providers have accessed their medical data and that no other doctor, nurse, or hospital has done so. In this way, while complete digital health records exist for every citizen, each knows that personal information belongs to them, neither to their doctor nor to the government.

This has made it easier to accept consolidated healthcare records and systems. After all, if your medical data is stored on paper files, you have far less control over who has read it than you do with digital records, where every reader leaves digital fingerprints. (If the system is adequately built, of course.)

Based on personal experience, I can testify that fully digital personal health records offer far superior patient experience to an alternative where each provider closely guards patient data. They say they do so for safety reasons, but in reality, they do so very often because of business interests. The risks related to integrated systems can be managed by adequate safeguarding and fire-walling methods. Since many paper-based systems have long used the data safety arguments in order not to transfer to digital ecosystems, considerable efforts may be needed to convince patients that digital healthcare records allow, in fact, better data protection and a superior level of personal control over sensitive health information.

A final warning - fragmented digital health systems that do not allow patients to transfer all their medical information - including pictures, analysis, etc. to the practitioner of their choice - will deliver neither savings nor satisfaction to patients. Therefore, digital healthcare systems must be designed to overcome the fragmented nature of many healthcare provision models! Even if it is in the business interests of hospitals and practitioners not to share the results of tests they ordered for their patients, the law must be clear that these results belong to the patient, not to the hospital. Therefore, they must be fully accessible via digital data systems to other providers if the patient wishes.

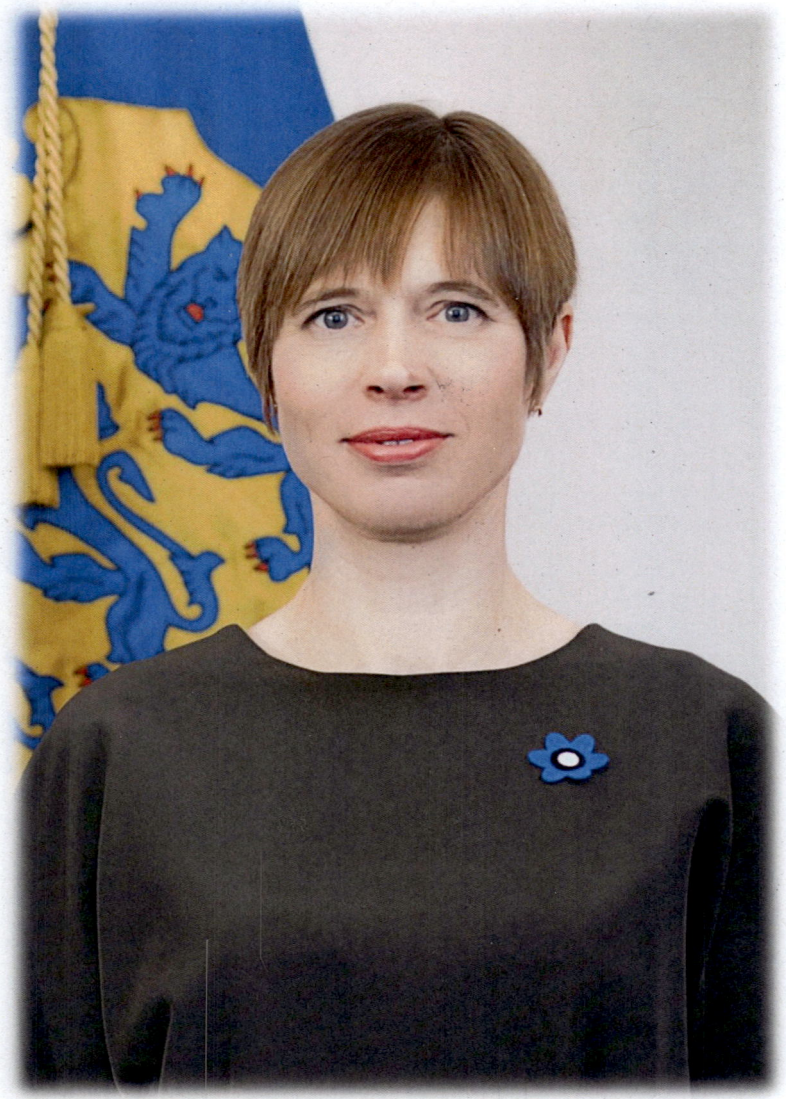

Figure 1. President Kersti Kaljulaid, Fifth President of Estonia (2016-2021)

PREFACE

In 2009, a political controversy surprised politicians who thought they were making a sensible suggestion. "Patients would be encouraged to store their medical records with companies like Google and Microsoft under plans being drawn up by the Conservatives." Using successful technology efforts by private companies seemed sensible, following the UK government's previous failed centralised effort with medical records. But the public backlash was immediate and sustained.

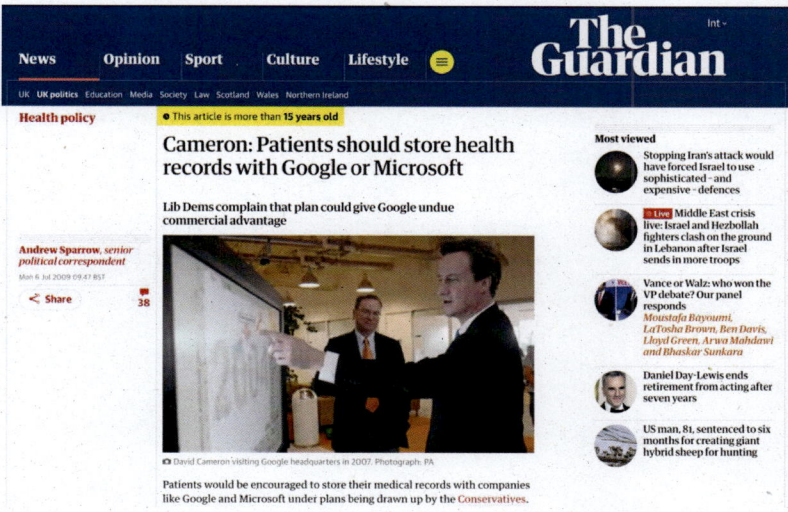

Figure 2. Controversy when the UK's Prime Minister recommended US tech companies' personal health records (The Guardian 2009)

The government quickly shelved the suggestion. Fifteen years later, the Labour government's Wes Streeting is using the same language about a single record for the citizen for life (The Guardian 2024). His new name is for "patient passport," and it would be integrated into the government-owned NHS App. However, he does not provide details on how to achieve this.

We see this dilemma facing every country. They need this technology, their citizens need this technology, and everyone needs it done right, right now. But governments do not know how to build, and they do not know how to buy.

We wrote this book to get governments past thinking and into acting. Most know why, few know what, and far too few know how. We wanted to document the experience of every country to advance every nation. Every citizen needs this.

Why personal health records?

In England, 1 in 17 people has a rare disease (Donaldson, 2010): most of these people know more about their situation than most of the doctors looking after them. 25-50% of patients at hospitals are from outside the region (Patients Know Best research 2024): the hospital does not have access to the records from outside the region. Long-term conditions account for about 70% of the money the country spends on health and social care (Nuffield Trust, 2024): what these patients do matters more than what their doctors do.

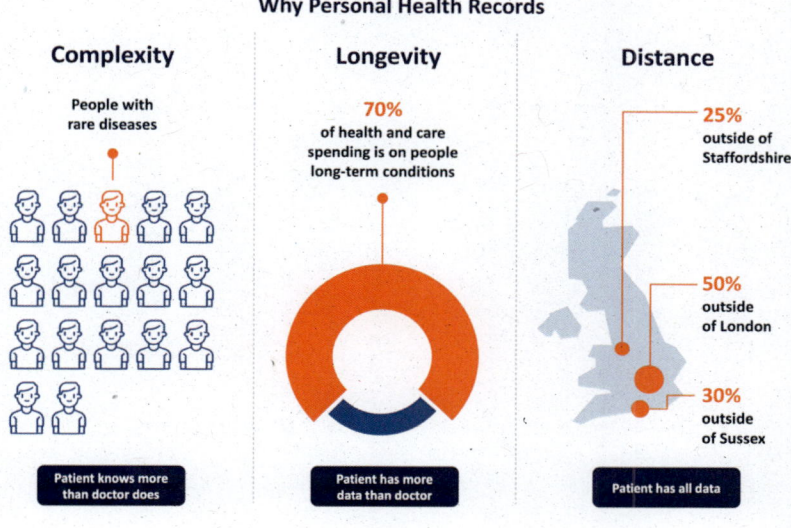

Figure 3

These three are the drivers for a health record that is organised around the person. A personal health record. This recognises the patient's knowledge, starting with rare disease patients. The record moves with the person, as expensive patients travel long distances to hospitals. And daily data from the person's body and actions determine health and death more than a hospital's episodic data.

Why governments?

Governments account for the majority of health care spending in the majority of countries. In the UK, the publicly owned National Health Service has long dominated, accounting for 80% of health care spending. Government spending still dominates countries with a majority of private providers. Even in the USA, public health spending was 52% pre-Covid in 2019 (up from 44% in 2000) (World Bank, 2024)—the trend of increasing government funding accelerated during Covid.

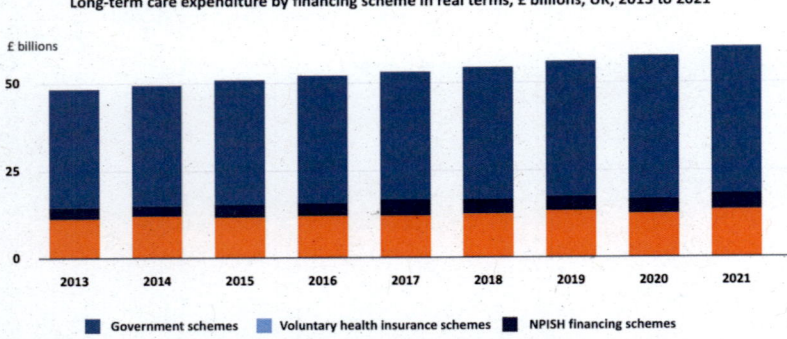

Total long-term care expenditure predominantly consisted of government spending in 2021

Long-term care expenditure by financing scheme in real terms, £ billions, UK, 2013 to 2021

Figure 4. Source : Office of National Statistics 2021

Governments are the insurers of last resort. They are the only ones taking on actuarial risk, socialising the risk of health care costs. Governments - not private insurers - are the ones covering rare diseases, long distances, and chronic conditions.

Therefore, it is governments that lead the process of personal health records. Private providers build organisational portals that lock in the patient to lock in the profits. Private payers' investments in portals stop when the member changes payer, and the member knows this, so they do not engage. Only the government has a financial incentive, at scale, over decades, to organise data around a citizen's lifetime.

Governments often start with government-owned providers: the Department of Veterans Affairs in the USA went first and farthest in personal health records, while private providers focused on organisational portals. Across Europe and the Gulf, public providers carried out data-sharing instructions first and faithfully. In India, public providers are the sleeping giant that will likely transform the percentage of data shared in structured, coded format rather than the current scanned, unstructured, uncoded PDFs of private providers.

Why now?

No government can deliver universal coverage in the 21st century without personal health records. As people with rare, distant, and complex situations live longer, their care is unaffordable if professionals do everything. Not every patient can do everything, but many can do much, and they must be allowed to.

Yet every government is expected to contribute more for universal coverage.

The share of government contribution is highest in the countries with the highest incomes. As countries' incomes rise, so does their government share. And high-income countries' government share has increased with time.

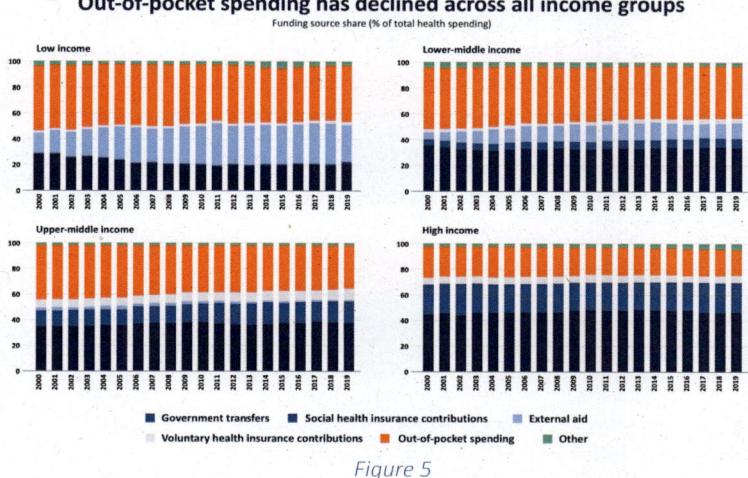

Figure 5

COVID-19 cemented this trend.

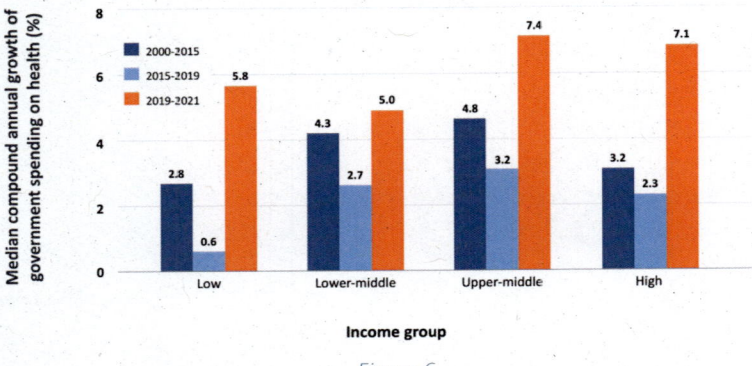

Government spending on health grew faster during the COVID-19 pandemic than during the Millennium Development Goals period and between the adoption of the Sustainable Development Goals and the pandemic

Figure 6

Therefore, every government must find a solution for the personal health records of its population.

Why the book?

Yet governments do not know how to solve this problem. They lack the skills to build, and they lack the trust to buy. They understand that personal health records are critical infrastructure for the 21st century, so they are fearful of making mistakes. Many build limited, idiosyncratic national solutions.

This is a good starting point. It is a long way from the destination. They start with transparency: a promise by the government to its citizens that data about the person will be visible to the person.

The private sector delivers engagement: driven by competition, a focus on usability means more people look at more data more quickly.

Activation is the goal: a citizen who understands what is happening and knows what to do about it. It will take a globally competitive industry of solutions to deliver this, just as the internet delivered two decades ago in other industries.

The goal of this book is to raise the game of governments. By documenting the efforts of different countries, officials can learn from each other more quickly. It is also to tilt trust as some governments have worked with the private sector, and some of those efforts have worked. We all must deliver activated citizens. There is no time to lose: the demands of aging, obesity, and workforce are crushing health systems; meanwhile, the advances in sensors and AI are astonishing.

This book is to seize the opportunity and dodge the disaster for the health of humankind.

Bibliography

- Donaldson, S.L. (2010) Preface. In: Department of Health, 2009 annual report of the Chief Medical Officer. Available at: http://www.sthc.co.uk/Documents/CMO_Report_2009.pdf (accessed: 26 August 2024).

- The Guardian 2009: Patients should store their health records with Google or Microsoft, says David Cameron (accessed: 29 October 2024).

- The Guardian 2024: Wes Streeting unveils plans for 'patient passports' to hold all medical records (accessed: 29 October 2024).

- Nuffield Trust (2024) Care and support for long term conditions. Available at: Care and support for long term conditions (accessed: 26 August 2024).

- Office of National Statistics 2021: Healthcare expenditure, UK Health Accounts - Office for National Statistics (accessed: 29 October 2024).

- World Bank (2024) Global Health Expenditure database. Available at: World Bank Open Data (accessed: 26 August 2024).

- World Health Organization (2023): Global spending on health: coping with the pandemic. Available at: https://iris.who.int/bitstream/handle/10665/375855/9789240086746-eng.pdf?sequence=1 (accessed: 29 October 2024).

SOURCES

Our sources include academic literature, newspaper articles, and information from government and corporate websites. Individuals worldwide were kind enough to log in and show us their data in their national systems. They are the source of screenshots in the book. Key figures involved in developing and implementing PHRs provided detailed historical context, often off the record.

All errors are ours as authors. The complexity of the subject and the dynamic research mean we will always have errors, and this book is an incomplete resource. Our commitment is to keep up with the rapidly evolving technologies discussed in the book, striving to provide a representation that closely mirrors reality.

To achieve this goal, we ask for your help: contact us to correct us at book@phr4gov.org.

INTRODUCTION

What Is a Personal Health Record?

Some History

A 1956 paper in the *Journal of the American Medical Association* proposed the idea of a 'personal health log' as a durable booklet that individuals should possess throughout their lives (Dragstedt, 1956). This 'personal health record' (PHR) was, therefore, a basic form of documentation containing essential health information for individuals to stay informed about their well-being.

Early investigations show that PHRs were often just a simple form of written notes containing the basic information a patient needs to know about their health. So, the importance of maintaining such records predates the digital age. Such records were variously called 'personal records,' 'personal health records, 'card files for personal record keeping,' and more (Kim et al.,2011). These records were basic because, previously, the medical service system and healthcare providers were the guardians of medical knowledge.

Today, the terms 'patient-held health records' and even 'personally-held health records' show the shift towards a more patient-centred approach in medicine. Healthcare consumers are generally now the main authorities in their health management.

The graph below shows the number of 'personal health record' publications per year from 1956 to 2023.

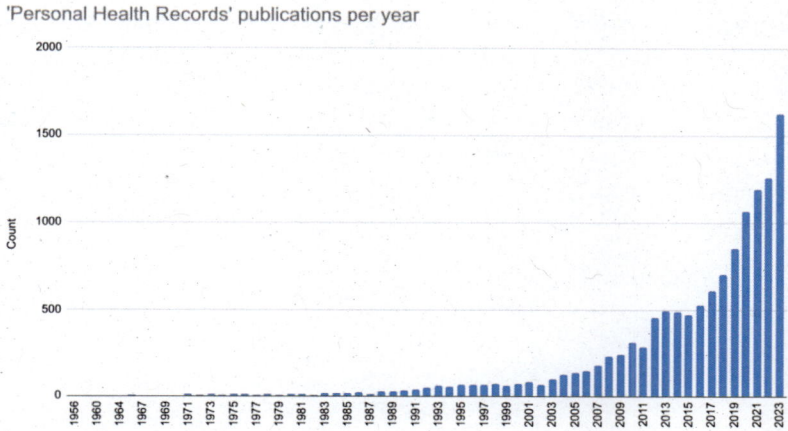

'Personal Health Records' publications per year

Figure 7. Number of personal health records publications per year (PubMed).

So, how is a PHR defined today? There is a lack of consensus about the standard definition, and the term is sometimes used to refer to any platform storing health data. For this book, PHRs have specific characteristics and should not be confused with patient-facing digital systems. In the next few paragraphs, we'll list some of the currently most used terms and explain their meaning.

Digital Systems

Authors use different definitions in different contexts, and fashions of definitions change over time. For the rest of this book, we will use the following definitions of the terms. For our purposes, the main difference between PHRs and other systems is the party that ultimately controls the record.

Electronic Health Record (EHR)

This is a digital version of a healthcare provider's paper chart. It is used by healthcare professionals only. Patients cannot access data in an EHR.

Tethered - Patient Portal (PP)

A **patient portal** gives a patient access to medical data but not ultimate control over access. If the patient controls access to the data, it is a PHR, a true personal health record ([Al-Ubaydli, 2011](#)). If the organisation controls it, it is an organisation portal. If a regional organisation controls it, it is an organisational portal, and so on.

Tethered Portals
create even more fragmentation

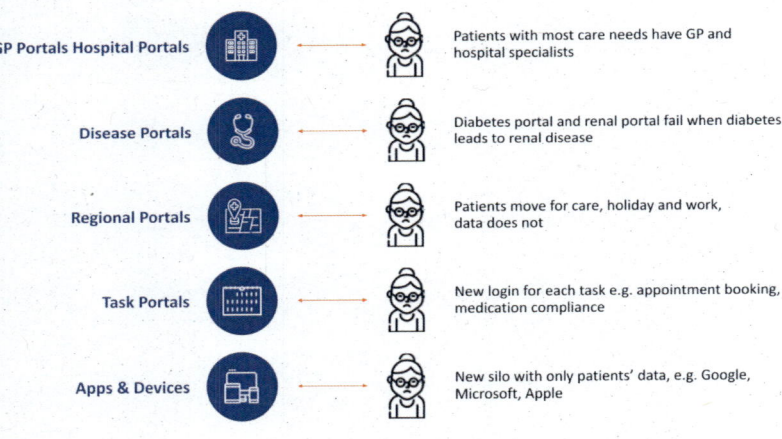

GP Portals Hospital Portals	Patients with most care needs have GP and hospital specialists
Disease Portals	Diabetes portal and renal portal fail when diabetes leads to renal disease
Regional Portals	Patients move for care, holiday and work, data does not
Task Portals	New login for each task e.g. appointment booking, medication compliance
Apps & Devices	New silo with only patients' data, e.g. Google, Microsoft, Apple

Figure 8

Therefore, patient portals include:

Organisational portals are patient portals that only show data from one organisation. For example, a GP portal shows data from the general practitioner of the patient, and a hospital portal shows data from the hospital. Access is ultimately under the control of the organisation.

Disease portals focus on a single condition, such as kidney disease or diabetes. They allow patients to record and monitor health data specific to this disease. The workflow and features are tailored to that disease. The main drawback of this focus is ignoring the other conditions the patients might have, including common conditions and commonly correlated ones (comorbidities). For example, people with diabetes often develop kidney disease. These diseases might be linked and interfere with the one the system is focusing on. This is a step back from a holistic view of patient health.

Regional portals: Some systems collect data from the EHRs in a specific area or region. These can be very effective as they bring together patients' data from local healthcare providers. However, they prevent data traveling when a patient travels. And they usually cannot cope with data from the patient's device.

Device Apps are apps where the only data source is a single device, such as a Fitbit. Patient-centered apps are apps where the only data source is data manually entered by the patients themselves.

Untethered - Personal Health Record (PHR)

This is similar to a patient portal, but it's managed and maintained by individuals. People can access, manage, and share the health information found in this record.

A PHR is a patient-centered digital health record. The person ultimately controls access to the record.

Here, we have an umbrella term for patient portals, tethered portals, versus part of untethered PHRs. It enables a two-way exchange of health information between patients and the healthcare system.

How do We Define a PHR?

Hopefully, it is now clear that a personal health record is an electronic collection of health documentation that the patient controls and maintains.

17

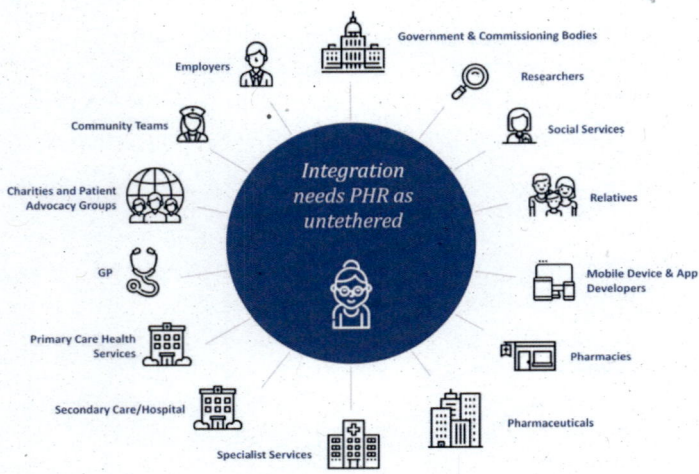

Figure 9

Patients can access their PHRs online and view test results, prescriptions, allergies, and other data from multiple EHRs. The individual can add to and update the record alongside the professionally-entered data.

With PHRs, a patient has a single, aggregated record that integrates data about them and follows them wherever they receive care. It's not locked to a particular geography, clinical system, organisation, or device.

Why Use PHRs?

Personal health records (PHRs) have the potential to revolutionise the way patients engage with the healthcare system and manage their health. They can be used to empower patients throughout the entire health cycle, from prevention to diagnosis, through treatment and recovery.

Advantages for Patients

Patients can self-assess and self-manage with a PHR. They can also receive safer and faster care when a professional assesses and manages them as the professional sees data from all care providers throughout the patient's life stages.

During the prevention phase, PHRs can provide patients with access to reliable and up-to-date information about how to prevent common illnesses and diseases. Patients can use PHRs to track their symptoms, measurements, and observations and then contact their doctors if they notice any anomalies.

During the **diagnostic** phase, PHRs can help patients track their symptoms and share them with their doctors. This can help speed up the diagnostic process and ensure patients receive the correct treatment.

During the **treatment** phase, PHRs assist patients in managing their conditions and tracking their progress. PHRs can also be used to monitor medication adherence and report any adverse reactions. In the case of surgery, PHRs can be used to provide patients with instructions for preparatory activities and to track post-op recovery.

During the **recovery** phase, PHRs can help patients monitor their progress and communicate with their healthcare providers. PHRs can also be used to facilitate patient-initiated follow-up, which can help ensure that patients receive the care they need.

Advantages for Professionals

With a PHR, professionals can treat more patients faster and safer. This is because the professional is more productive and because the patient can take on some of the work.

Since patient-professional alliances significantly influence health outcomes, empowering patients can potentially improve health.

PHRs give healthcare professionals access to a comprehensive overview of a patient's current health status and medical history. This enables them to make better-informed decisions regarding treatment and care plans. In turn, this increases the likelihood of treatment success.

PHRs help patients and healthcare professionals communicate electronically, making it easier and faster for them to connect, thereby improving communication. Using PHRs for patient communication has the potential to reduce the workload for professionals, as they can spend less time on phone calls and managing multiple inboxes. Moreover, effective message-based exchanges on the PHR platform may lead to fewer face-to-face consultations, as certain issues can be addressed through digital consultations.

Healthcare professionals' workload will also be decreased because the patients take on some of the more straightforward tasks like monitoring and recording their own blood pressure or blood glucose levels.

Advantages for Providers

With better records, providers can lower costs and increase revenue by attracting more patients.

When professionals are burdened with excessive administrative tasks, documentation, and other non-clinical work, their productivity and efficiency can be significantly impacted. The use of PHRs reduces this burden and can improve healthcare providers' efficiency in various ways:

Increased productivity and better patient care: Reduced administrative work frees up more time for professionals to focus on patient care activities, such as consultations, examinations, and treatments. This can lead to improved decision-making, patient outcomes, and satisfaction.

Enhanced job satisfaction: Professionals who are not burdened by administrative tasks often experience higher job satisfaction. This can result in lower turnover rates and a more stable healthcare workforce.

Improved collaboration: When professionals have more time, they can collaborate more effectively with colleagues. This can lead to better care coordination and improved patient outcomes.

By reducing the burden on professionals, healthcare organisations can improve overall provider efficiency and the quality of care they provide to patients.

Advantages for the Payer

There are multiple reasons why using PHRs benefits healthcare payors.

Prevention: PHRs enable individuals to take proactive steps to prevent illnesses, reducing the need for costly treatments in the future. They also enhance patient safety by identifying health risks early, again decreasing the need for major interventions later.

Self-monitoring:

- Patients who use PHRs to manage their health and wellness can reduce their healthcare costs by reducing the number of appointments they need.
- Informed patients make appointments more time-efficient.
- PHRs alleviate disruptions in treatment for chronic conditions.

- In general, patients who are self-monitoring through PHRs are less likely to have A&E admissions and surgeries. If they do need these, PHRs make emergency handling smoother.

Better medication adherence: PHRs help patients adhere to their medication regimens, resulting in better health outcomes and reduced healthcare costs.

Online appointment management: PHRs allow patients to manage their appointments online, reducing the number of DNA (Did Not Attend) appointments. This frees up space for other patients, improving overall healthcare efficiency.

In general, a country whose citizens can use a PHR will have a higher quality of care at lower costs.

In a research paper titled 'Utility, Value, and Benefits of Contemporary Personal Health Records: Integrative Review and Conceptual Synthesis,' Ruhi and Chugh (2021) summarised their findings in a table (Table 2) named 'Value Propositions and Benefits of Personal Health Record Systems to Health Care Delivery Constituents'.

Here are their findings:

Consumer empowerment and patient engagement

- Promote consumer health education
- Enable patients to become informed healthcare consumers
- Enhance understanding of medical conditions
- Simplify and clarify patient instructions
- Provide greater control over health outcomes
- Offer convenient self-health management
- Facilitate self-efficacy via cues for patient action

Healthcare communication

- Improve patient-physician or provider communication
- Timely information sharing for clinical decisions
- End-to-end care delivery involving multiple constituents

Process efficiencies and cost-effectiveness

- Increased patient records portability
- Reduced chronic disease management costs
- Greater medical information validity and accuracy
- Save patient, physician, and provider time
- Reduced cost of tests and procedures duplication

Enhanced quality of care

- Increased patient safety considerations
- Improved emergency situation handling
- Extended patient data durability
- Early identification of patient risks and health susceptibilities

Public health outcomes

- Reduced burden on the health care system and resources
- Enhanced care for underserved communities and populations
- Facilitate care in public health emergencies
- Support public health research
- New avenues for epidemiology surveillance and screening

Advantages for the Planet

PHRs have the potential to reduce carbon emissions in healthcare through:

- Replacing in-person patient appointments with remote interactions, thus avoiding carbon emissions from journeys to medical facilities.
- Allowing patients to remotely monitor themselves, thereby reducing unnecessary visits to the emergency department, admissions, and surgical procedures, all of which contribute to carbon emissions.
- Substituting paper records and letters with digital alternatives reduces deforestation, lowers waste, and decreases energy use for paper production. It also cuts down on carbon emissions from the transportation and storage of physical documents. This helps in reducing carbon emissions.

Challenges in Implementing a PHR

Change Resistance

Multiple studies have shown that implementing a new system in healthcare usually meets resistance. Also, they've shown that only a few medical workers embrace changes. Usually, healthcare workers face changes with distrust, doubts, and even rejection.

Payment models significantly increase the resistance to change in healthcare.

Healthcare professionals are typically compensated for specific tasks they perform. With the introduction of tools like PHR, patients can take on some of these tasks themselves. As a result, professionals may find themselves engaging in new activities that are not directly reimbursed while the patient takes over activities the professional was previously reimbursed for.

This gap between old payment systems and new roles makes it difficult to adopt and integrate changes.

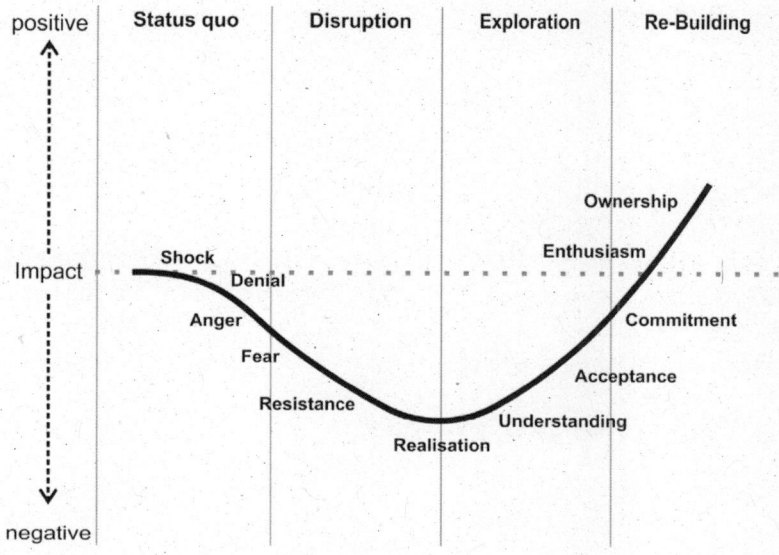

Figure 10. Model of the sequence of psychological conditions in a person dealing with a change they find threatening (based on the model by Kübler-Ross) (Mareš, 2018).

Training

One of the challenges in implementing the PHR system is the provision of adequate training. This refers to both current and future healthcare professionals' training.

Students' training: Studies show a lack of digital health in medical education. There's a gap between the willingness of medical students to become digital transformation leaders in healthcare and the education that they receive.

Healthcare professionals' training: Implementing a PHR successfully requires all the professionals involved to be trained on the system. Lack of training is one of the key barriers to PHR adoption.

Fragmentation

Developing and implementing a personal health record (PHR) presents the challenge of populating it with relevant data. Patients' health information is historically scattered across various healthcare institutions' information systems. Different systems hold parts of their medical history and current health status. This leads to fragmented medical data when patients receive treatment from multiple providers. PHRs are urgently needed to consolidate patients' complete medical records into one single record, addressing the significant challenge posed by this data fragmentation.

Additionally, workflow fragmentation occurs due to the presence of multiple systems within the same institution, including those for training and communication.

Bibliography

- Al-Ubaydli, M., 2011. Personal health records: a guide for clinicians. John Wiley & Sons. Available at: https://www.wiley.com/en-us/Personal+Health+Records%3A+A+Guide+for+Clinicians-p-9781444348255 (accessed: 3 November 2024).

- Dragstedt, C.A., 1956. Personal health log: guest editorial. Journal of the American Medical Association, 160(15), pp.1320-1320. Available at: https://doi.org/10.1001/jama.1956.02960500050013 (accessed: 3 November 2024).

- Kim, J., Jung, H. and Bates, D.W., 2011. History and Trends of. Healthcare informatics research, 17(1), pp.3-17. Available at: https://doi.org/10.4258/hir.2011.17.1.3 (accessed: 3 November 2024).

- Mareš, J., 2018. Resistance of health personnel to changes in healthcare. Kontakt, 20(3), pp.e262-e272. Available at: https://www.sciencedirect.com/science/article/abs/pii/S1212411718300114 (accessed: 3 November 2024).

- Ruhi, U. and Chugh, R., 2021. Utility, valxue, and benefits of contemporary personal health records: integrative review and conceptual synthesis. Journal of medical Internet research, 23(4), p.e26877. Available at: https://doi.org/10.2196/26877 (accessed: 3 November 2024).

DENMARK

Over half of the world's hearing aids are made by 3 Danish companies (UBS 2019). In 1950, Denmark became the first country in the world to provide free hearing aids to its citizens (Hindhede 2013). The country combines a comprehensive and generous government welfare system with an innovative and entrepreneurial private sector.

Country's healthcare system in a nutshell

Denmark's healthcare system is built on four pillars (Sternberg, 2022):

- Universal coverage
- Financed by general taxes
- Free and equal access
- High degree of decentralisation

The system has fully embraced digitalisation. Each region is responsible for storing electronic health record (EHR) data in the region's data repository. EHR coverage is comprehensive, with healthcare providers legally required to report to these regional repositories. The two EHR systems in use (EPIC and Systematic) operate independently without direct data exchange. The national E-Journal shows healthcare professionals information from the EHRs of other regions (Fragidis & Chatzoglou, 2018; Jensen & Thorseng, 2017; Tikkanen et al., 2020).

Health insurance covers the entire population of Denmark: both members of health insurance schemes and those with free access to state-provided healthcare services (Our World in Data, 2011).

Public vs private

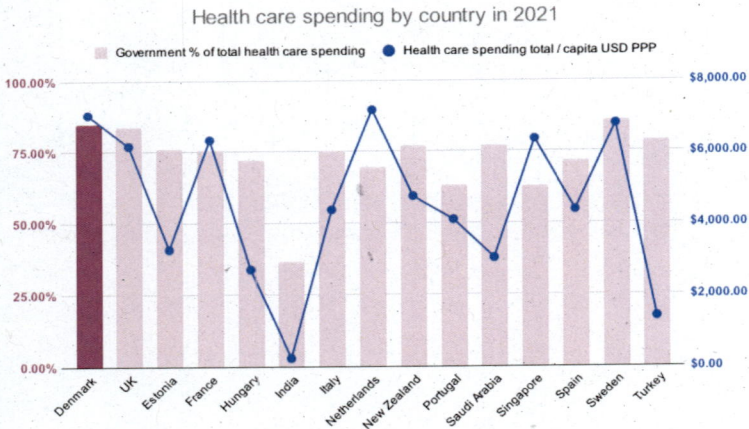

Figure 11. Source: The World Bank. The pink column refers to the public expenditure as a % of the country's total healthcare expenditure. The blue dot is the country's expenditure on health per capita, expressed in international dollars at purchasing power parity.

The national PHR

History

Sundhed.dk is a public, internet-based portal where every citizen can log in to see their medical records, and healthcare professionals can see their patients' records.

Sundhed.dk dates back to 2001, when a broad political governing body was formed to support the development of a national e-health portal. This body included the Association of County Councils, the Ministry of the Interior and Health, the Greater Capital's Hospital Association, and the municipalities of Copenhagen and Frederiksberg.

Sundhed.dk Timeline of Main Events

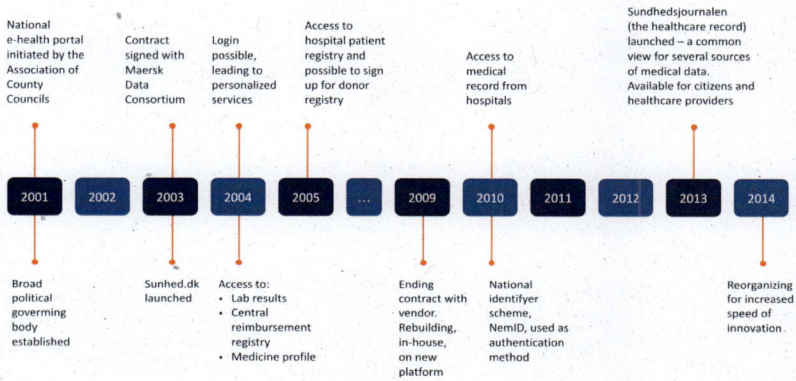

Figure 12. Timeline of main events (Jensen and Thorseng 2017 Fig 13.1).

Given the scale and complexity of building the shared infrastructure, the board of directors chose to conduct the tender as a competition in 2002. The Maersk Data Consortium—comprising LEC, ACURE, PLS/Ramboll, and Bysted—won the contest. The central office of Sundhed.dk signed a contract with the consortium in early 2003.

Patients did not gain access to their data until 2009.

In April 2009, Sundhed.dk was relaunched on a new technical platform, and an internal development department took over most of the service development, while external consultants were brought in only for standalone services—reversing the previous approach. One of the first initiatives at that time was to make medical records from public hospitals accessible to patients, allowing them to view parts of their records, such as treatments, diagnoses, and notes made by healthcare personnel (Jensen and Thorseng, 2017; Sundhed.dk, 2023).

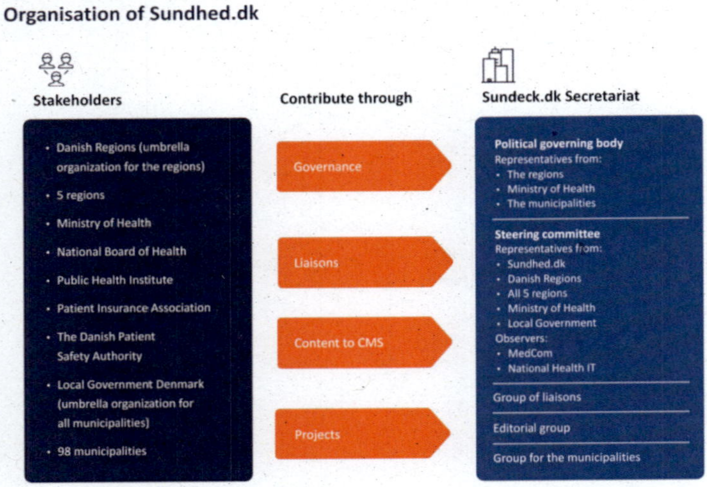

Organisation of Sundhed.dk

Figure 13. Organisation of Sundhed.dk (Jensen and Thorseng 2017 Fig 13.2)

Features

Sundhed.dk has a federated architecture. It draws from 120 local systems without storing or duplicating.

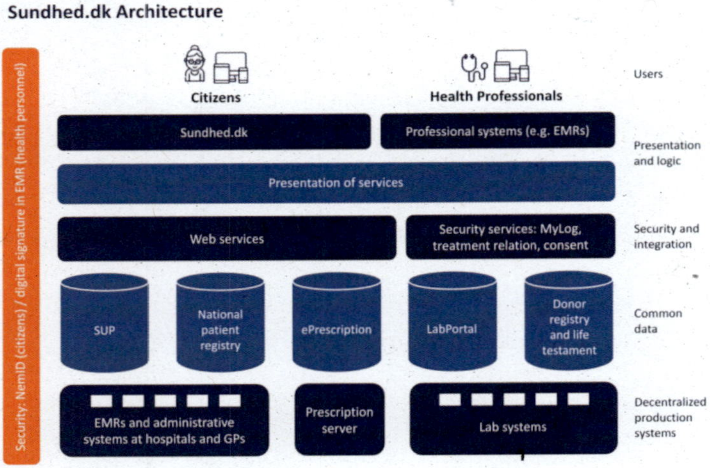

Sundhed.dk Architecture

Figure 14. (Jensen and Thorseng, 2017 Fig 13.3)

Patients can log in after identity verification. Their medical records include data from general practitioners (GPs), hospital electronic health record (EHR) systems (Petersen, 2019), and certain private health professionals (Hartlev, 2014). Features include (Sundhed.dk, 2023):

- Accessing their health journal with medical records from healthcare providers. Records include imaging reports, test results, referrals, discharge letters, medications, and vaccinations.
- Seeing past appointments with GPs, specialists, and public hospitals.
- Requesting repeat prescriptions.
- Registering or deregistering as an organ donor, creating a treatment will, checking the status of screening procedures, and granting relatives power of attorney to view their health data.
- Marking certain information as private to hide from healthcare professionals using Sundhed.dk. A hospital's employees can still see the data in their hospital's local EHR.

Healthcare professionals can access their patients' health data through Sundhed.dk. It also provides clinical information and guidelines that may not be available in their local EHR. For example, GPs can access hospital EHRs, waiting lists, and contact details for other healthcare professionals (Petersen, 2019).

Challenges and areas for improvement

Despite its many strengths, there are still areas where the system could improve to further enhance patient engagement and functionality.

- The inability of patients to connect personal health devices, such as home monitoring devices, to their records.

- Patients cannot currently add their own health data to their medical records.

Statistics

Usage

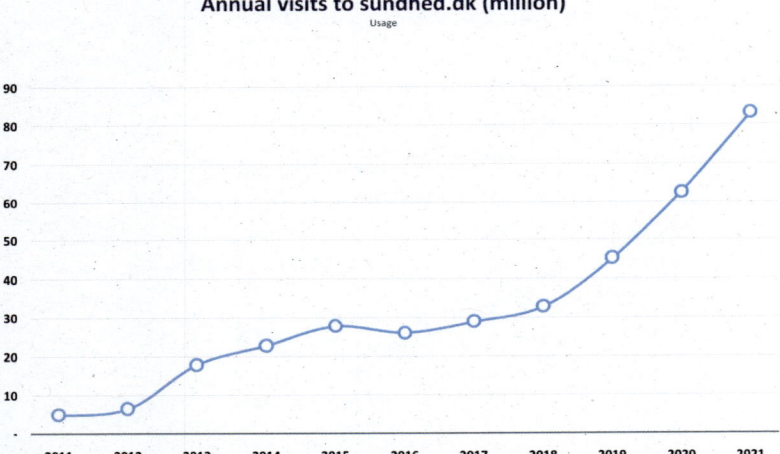

Annual visits to sundhed.dk (million)
Usage

Figure 15. The Norwegian Directorate of eHealth, 2022

Most used services

- Laboratory results (Corona test results included).
- Patient journal.
- Medicine card.
- Patient & Doctors handbook.
- Image descriptions.
- Appointments.
- Find a practitioner.

([The Norwegian Directorate of eHealth, 2022](#))

Nordics NPS and knowledge

Net Promoter Score (NPS) is a tool to measure customer likelihood of recommending a company, a product, or a service to a friend or colleague.

- -100-0: Bad
- 0-30: Good
- 30-70: Very good
- 70-100: Excellent

Denmark:

- Net Promoter Score: 21 (2021)
- 96% have heard of sundhed.dk (2021)

In comparison to other Northern European countries for context:

Finland:

- Net Promoter Score*: 52 (2020)
- Second most respected website (2020)

Norway:

- Net Promoter Score*: 48 (2021)
- 97% have heard of Helsenorge (2021)

Sweden:

- Net Promoter Score*: 45 (2021)
- 99% have heard of 1177 (2020)

(The Norwegian Directorate of eHealth, 2022)

Screenshots

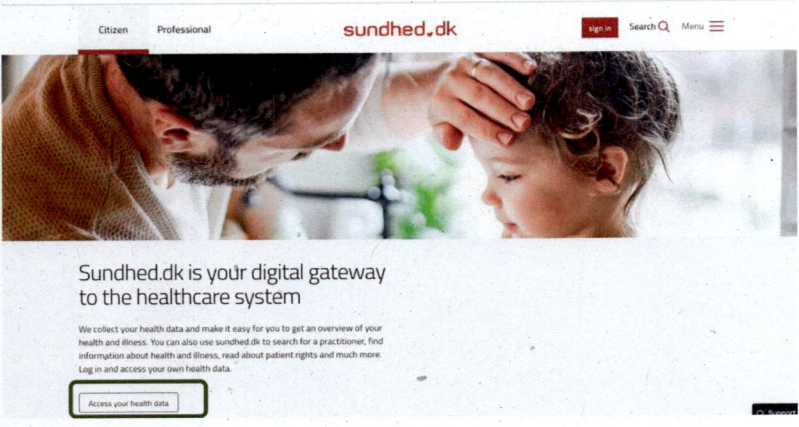

Figure 16. Homepage of Sundhed.dk

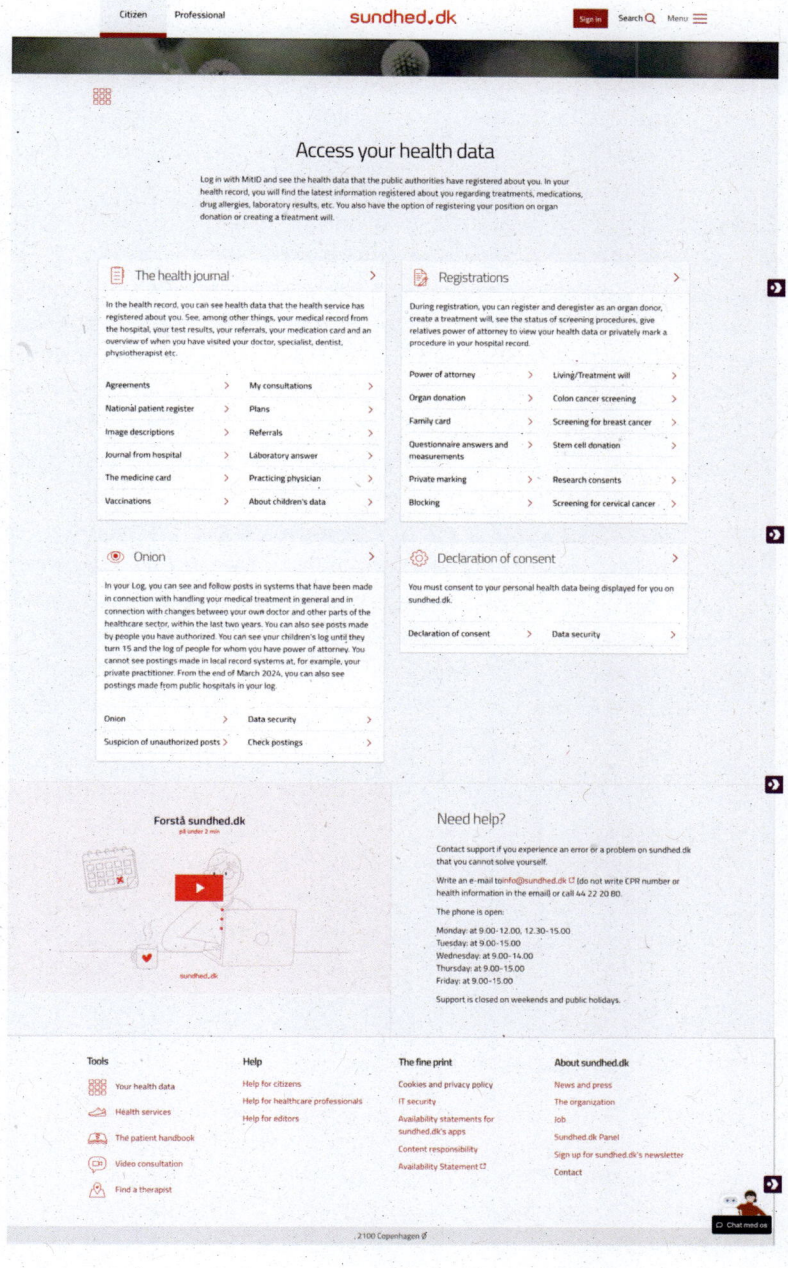

Citizen   Professional

sundhed.dk

Sign in   Search 🔍   Menu ☰

Access your health data

Log in with MitID and see the health data that the public authorities have registered about you. In your health record, you will find the latest information registered about you regarding treatments, medications, drug allergies, laboratory results, etc. You also have the option of registering your position on organ donation or creating a treatment will.

📄 The health journal   ›

In the health record, you can see health data that the health service has registered about you. See, among other things, your medical record from the hospital, your test results, your referrals, your medication card and an overview of when you have visited your doctor, specialist, dentist, physiotherapist etc.

Agreements	›	My consultations	›
National patient register	›	Plans	›
Image descriptions	›	Referrals	›
Journal from hospital	›	Laboratory answer	›
The medicine card	›	Practicing physician	›
Vaccinations	›	About children's data	›

📝 Registrations   ›

During registration, you can register and deregister as an organ donor, create a treatment will, see the status of screening procedures, give relatives power of attorney to view your health data or privately mark a procedure in your hospital record.

Power of attorney	›	Living/Treatment will	›
Organ donation	›	Colon cancer screening	›
Family card	›	Screening for breast cancer	›
Questionnaire answers and measurements	›	Stem cell donation	›
Private marking	›	Research consents	›
Blocking	›	Screening for cervical cancer	›

◎ Onion   ›

In your Log, you can see and follow posts in systems that have been made in connection with handling your medical treatment in general and in connection with changes between your own doctor and other parts of the healthcare sector, within the last two years. You can also see posts made by people you have authorized. You can see your children's log until they turn 15 and the log of people for whom you have power of attorney. You cannot see postings made in local record systems at, for example, your private practitioner. From the end of March 2024, you can also see postings made from public hospitals in your log.

Onion	›	Data security	›
Suspicion of unauthorized posts	›	Check postings	›

⚙ Declaration of consent   ›

You must consent to your personal health data being displayed for you on sundhed.dk.

Declaration of consent	›	Data security	›

Forstå sundhed.dk
på under 2 min

sundhed.dk

Need help?

Contact support if you experience an error or a problem on sundhed.dk that you cannot solve yourself.

Write an e-mail to info@sundhed.dk ⬈ (do not write CPR number or health information in the email) or call 44 22 20 80.

The phone is open:

Monday: at 9.00-12.00, 12.30-15.00
Tuesday: at 9.00-15.00
Wednesday: at 9.00-14.00
Thursday: at 9.00-15.00
Friday: at 9.00-15.00

Support is closed on weekends and public holidays.

Tools	Help	The fine print	About sundhed.dk
Your health data	Help for citizens	Cookies and privacy policy	News and press
Health services	Help for healthcare professionals	IT security	The organization
The patient handbook	Help for editors	Availability statements for sundhed.dk's apps	Job
Video consultation		Content responsibility	Sundhed.dk Panel
Find a therapist		Availability Statement ⬈	Sign up for sundhed.dk's newsletter
			Contact

2100 Copenhagen Ø

💬 Chat med os

This screenshot shows what patients see after selecting "Access your health data" on Sundhed. The original Danish translation contains some inaccuracies. Here's the revised version: The "Access your health data" section allows patients to log in with MitID to view health data that the healthcare sector has recorded about them. The "Health journal" provides access to hospital records, test results, referrals, the patient's medication card, and a summary of past visits to general practitioners, specialists, dentists, and physiotherapists. "Laboratory answers" should be corrected to "Laboratory results," and "Practicing physician" should be revised to "General practitioner." The "Declaration of Consent" requires patients to give consent for their personal health data to be displayed on Sundhed.dk. In the "Registrations" section, the phrase "status of screening procedures" should be changed to "Status of screening process." Additionally, "Onion" should be corrected to "Log," where patients can view and track inquiries made by systems regarding their medical treatment and transitions between healthcare providers over the past two years. This log also shows inquiries made by individuals who have been granted power of attorney, and patients can view their children's logs until they turn 15, as well as those of individuals for whom they hold power of attorney.

Bibliography

- Fragidis, L.L. and Chatzoglou, P.D., 2018. Implementation of a nationwide electronic health record (EHR): The international experience in 13 countries. International Journal of Health Care Quality Assurance, 31(2), pp.116-130. Available at: https://www.emerald.com/insight/content/doi/10.1108/IJHCQA-09-2016-0136/full/html (accessed: 3 November 2024).

- Hartlev, M., 2014. Overview of the national laws on electronic health records in the EU Member States: National Report for Denmark. Available at: https://health.ec.europa.eu/document/download/adaaa3b6-b336-4e65-8897-2b05a689f193_en (accessed: 21 August 2024).

- Hindhede, A and Larsen, K, 2019. The rise and fall of audiology in Denmark, 1950-2010. Available at https://prakti-skegrunde.dk/2013/praktiskegrunde(2013-1+2f)hindhede-larsen.pdf (accessed: 2 November 2024).

- Jensen, T.B. and Thorseng, A.A., 2017. Building national healthcare infrastructure: the case of the Danish e-health portal. In Information Infrastructures within European Health Care: Working with the Installed Base, pp.209-224. Available at: https://www.ncbi.nlm.nih.gov/books/NBK543679/ (accessed: 25 July 2024).

- Nielsen, N.B., Sekkal, C.K. and Yoganathan, S., 2021. Online Investigations on Optimizing the Danish Health Portal Sundhed.dk. In Context Sensitive Health Informatics: The Role of Informatics in Global Pandemics, pp.89-93. IOS Press. Available at: https://ebooks.iospress.nl/doi/10.3233/SHTI210644 (accessed: 3 November 2024).

- Our World in Data, 2011. Percentage of population covered by health insurance. Available at: https://our-worldindata.org/grapher/health-protection-coverage (accessed: 2 November 2024).

- Petersen, M.E., 2019. Achieving better health and well-being via the Danish e-Health portal sundhed.dk. Eurohealth, 25(2), pp.20-23. Available at: https://iris.who.int/bitstream/han-dle/10665/332595/Eurohealth-25-2-20-23-eng.pdf (accessed: 25 July 2024).

- Sternberg, J., 2022. Denmark: the leading digital health nation. Digital Switzerland. Available at: https://digitalswitzerland.com/den-mark-the-leading-digital-health-nation-a-magical-country/ (accessed: 25 July 2024).

- Sundhed.dk, 2023. Background. Available at: https://www.sundhed.dk/borger/service/om-sundheddk/om-organ-isationen/ehealth-in-denmark/background/ (accessed: 25 July 2024).

- TEHDAS Towards European Health Data Space, n.d. TEHDAS country visits. Available at: https://tehdas.eu/tehdas1/packages/package-4-

outreach-engagement-and-sustainability/tehdas-country-visits/ (accessed: 25 July 2024).

- The Norwegian Directorate of eHealth, 2022. Comparative analysis 2022: National Health Portals in the Nordics. Available at: https://assets.ctfassets.net/e03pgm1m5c6m/32Ntg6PRQXKIKjuCHpGKBU/cb0a883fb7b0bd651f71b9ef68da1cd9/2022_Nordic_National_Health_Portals_report_v1.1__1_.pdf (accessed: 25 July 2024).

- Tikkanen, R., Osborn, R., Mossialos, E., Djordjevic, A. and Wharton, G.A., 2020. International Health Care System Profiles - Denmark. The Commonwealth Fund. Available at: https://www.commonwealthfund.org/international-health-policy-center/countries/denmark (accessed: 25 July 2024).

- Towart, L. and Meyer, S.R., 2019. Longer term investments: medical devices. UBS. Available at:https://www.ubs.com/content/dam/WealthManagementAmericas/cio-impact/Medical Devices.pdf (accessed: 2 November 2024).

ENGLAND

Welfare more than offset the deaths from warfare in England. The most considerable improvements in life expectancy happened during the decades of WWI and WWII because of the government's increase in welfare (Preston, 1972). And in 1948, the UK created the National Health Service.

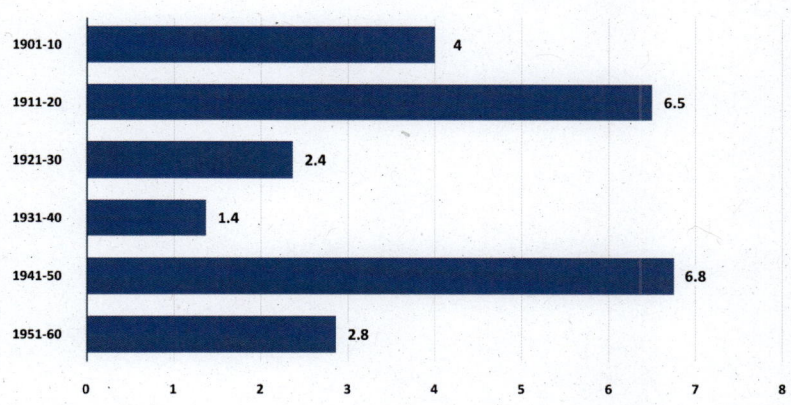

Improvements in life expectancy in England and Wales, 1901-1960

Figure 17. Preston, 1972.

Country's healthcare system in a nutshell

In the United Kingdom, the National Health Service (NHS) provides publicly funded universal healthcare coverage (Our World in Data, n.p.), along with publicly funded care providers. Every individual is required to register with a primary care general practitioner (GP). GP appointments are free of charge, and access to secondary care typically requires a GP referral.

Healthcare is devolved to each of the four nations of the United Kingdom, with NHS England serving the largest population of 58 million people. England separated government-owned providers from government-funded payers, while Scotland (5.5 million), Wales (3 million), and Northern Ireland (2 million) did not.

Despite the dominance of the public system, private healthcare options, as well as various alternative and complementary treatments, are available to those who can afford them (European Observatory on Health Systems and Policies, 2022).

Public vs private

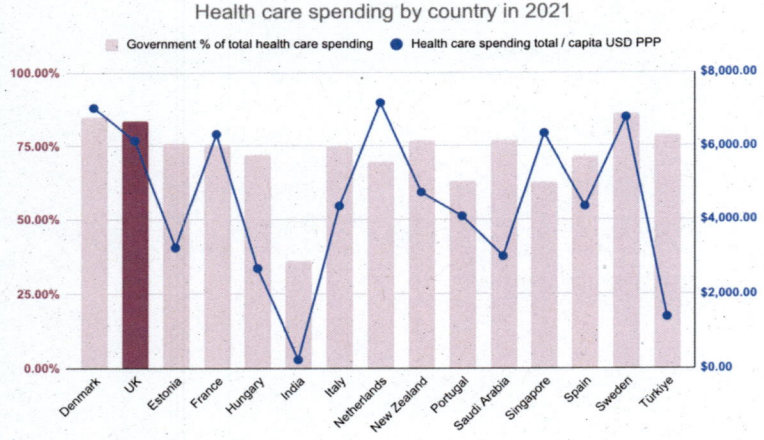

Figure 18. Source: The World Bank. The pink column refers to the public expenditure as a % of the country's total healthcare expenditure. The blue dot is the country's expenditure on health per capita, expressed in international dollars at purchasing power parity.

The national portal

History

NHS England's NHS App's 2019 launch was a significant milestone in the modernisation of the National Health Service. Developed collaboratively by NHSX, NHS Digital, and NHS England, the project got support from Health Ministers Jeremy Hunt and Matt Hancock, who both saw the app as a force driving technological advancement within the NHS.

Launch

Eight fundamental patient care challenges in 2017 drove the Secretary of State's investment in the NHS App, from symptom checking and triage to facilitating end-of-life care choices. Additionally, the app aimed to facilitate administrative tasks such as booking GP appointments, ordering repeat prescriptions, and managing data sharing and organ donation preferences.

The pilot phase began in October 2018 in regions including Liverpool, Staffordshire, Redditch, Bromsgrove, and others. During this phase, the app provided essential functions such as symptom checking, appointment booking, prescription orders, and access to patient records.

From 2019, it was planned that the app would support GP video consultations and integrate with wearable devices like the Apple Watch and Fitbit. These have not yet been developed and are in future roadmaps. Future integration with the NHS e-Referral Service will allow patients to book hospital or clinic appointments.

By January 2019, the app was available for download, though each GP practice needed to release data and appointment slots. This functionality was enabled through direct contracts between NHS

England, GP providers, and GP software companies, shaping the app's delivery focus (Bostock, 2019).

The NHS login provided a robust identity verification system. Patients could do this remotely without taking up clinical time or waiting.

Expansion

The app should not have additional features but instead serve as a platform for others to innovate on top of. NHSX CEO stated this in 2019 (Duffy, 2020). NHSX was established as the central IT department for the NHS.

In 2020, Patients Know Best (PKB) became the first Personal Health Record (PHR) to integrate with the NHS App. It included PKB's full health and care records and functionality.

COVID-19 Pass

Starting on 17 May 2021, the NHS App began displaying COVID-19 vaccination records, initially to support international travel. Over the following months, this feature evolved into the "NHS COVID Pass." Lockdowns significantly increased the use and adoption of the NHS App.

Monthly New NHS App Downloads and Registrations

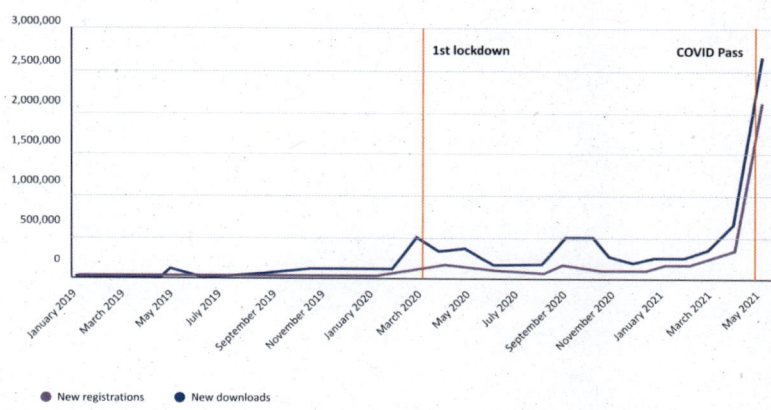

Figure 19. Monthly new NHS App downloads and registrations. Kc et al. (2023) 'Uptake and adoption of the NHS App in England,' British Journal of General Practice, 73(737), pp. e932–e940.

PEPs vs PHRs

In 2022, NHS England introduced the term Patient Engagement Platform (PEP). As NHS England's starting focus was administrative, the first PEP procurements focused on hospital appointment management features. Next were letter display and questionnaire completion features.

NHS England is expanding its focus on clinical usage, releasing clinical data to deliver clinical transformation. This functionality relies on PHRs.

Features

England is the only country identified in this research that has successfully created a marketplace for healthcare innovation through the NHS App.

NHS England achieved this by integrating private companies' features into its public platform. This has created a competitive environment where private developers are incentivized to develop high-quality, innovative solutions that meet the needs of NHS patients ([Al-Ubaydli, 2024](#)).

The NHS App has, therefore, three sets of functionality:

- National functionality, paid for and built through central government funding. This was the starting point of the NHS App in 2019.
- GP-commissioned functionality determined extra features each patient sees, i.e., functionality their GP surgery had chosen for all the patients in that surgery. This was the initial marketplace of electronic consultation systems and personal health records.
- Secondary care-commissioned PEP features. Each patient sees additional functionality that their hospital has bought for the patients treated at that hospital. This use interface is organised around appointments, starting with administration features and expanding to clinical features.

This page shows all the organisations, their corresponding product, and their functionality that have integrated with the NHS App: https://digital.nhs.uk/services/nhs-app/how-to-integrate-with-the-nhs-app/nhs-app-integrated-partners-and-services

Core national functionality

The core national functionality allows patients to interact with their GP's electronic health record system, including the ability to:

- Order repeat prescriptions.
- Nominate a pharmacy for prescription collection.
- Book and manage appointments.

- View their GP health record, including information such as allergies and medications.
- Book and manage COVID-19 vaccinations.
- Access their NHS COVID Pass.
- Register their organ donation decision.
- Choose how the NHS uses their GP data.
- View their NHS number.

Screenshots of core NHS App functionality:

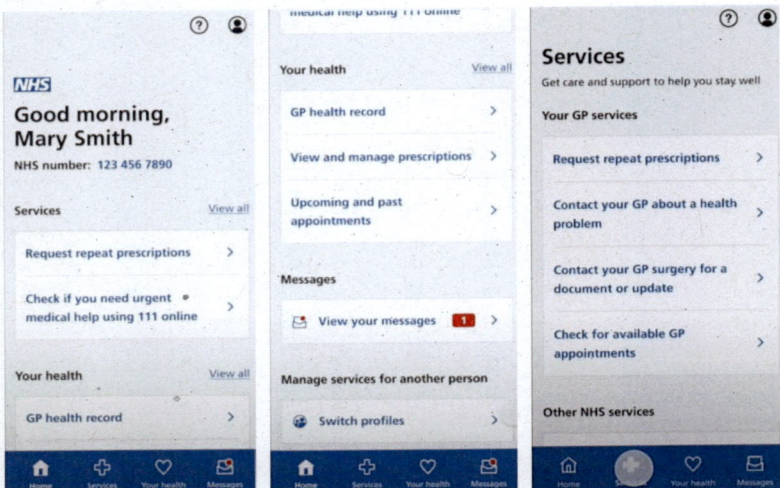

Figure 20. The homepage includes shortcuts to some of the most used areas of the NHS App. For example, patients can request repeat prescriptions and use 111 online.

Figure 21. Other shortcuts on the homepage include viewing their GP health record, viewing and managing prescriptions, as well as upcoming and past appointments. Patients can also see their messages and switch profiles to see the NHS App account of a relative or a person they care for.

Figure 22. The 'Services' page includes requesting repeat prescriptions, contacting their GP about a health problem, contacting their GP surgery for a document or update, and checking for available GP appointments.

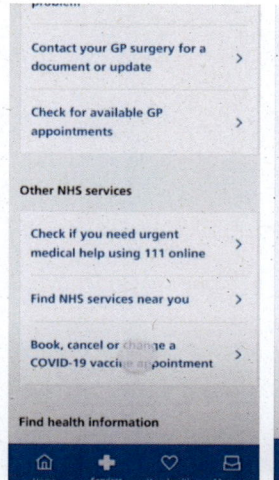

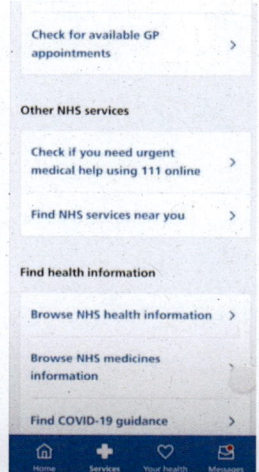

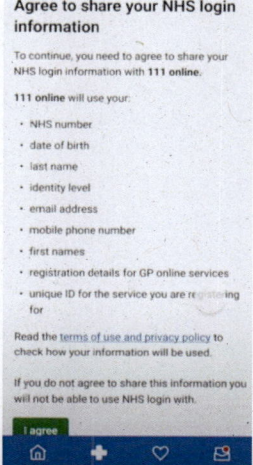

Figure 23. Other services include using 111 online, finding NHS services near them, and booking, canceling, or changing a COVID-19 vaccine appointment.

Figure 24. Lastly, services include browsing trusted NHS health and medicines information, as well as finding COVID-19 guidance. Some of these services depend on the GP surgery, so not all patients will see all of these options.

Figure 25. When using the 111 online service, patients are asked to agree to give certain information to the online service.

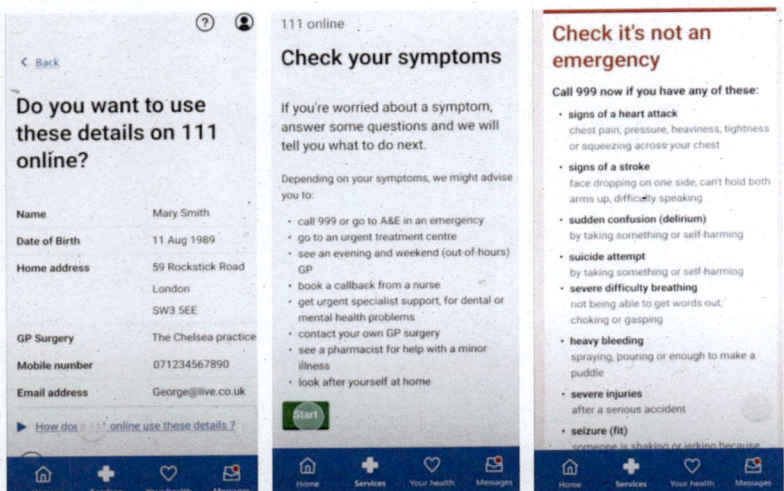

Figure 26. Patients can then check whether their details are correct.

Figure 27. Patients can then read more information on the functioning of the service and click start.

Figure 28. The app then presents a list of symptoms the patients must check. If any of these symptoms are present, the patient should call 999.

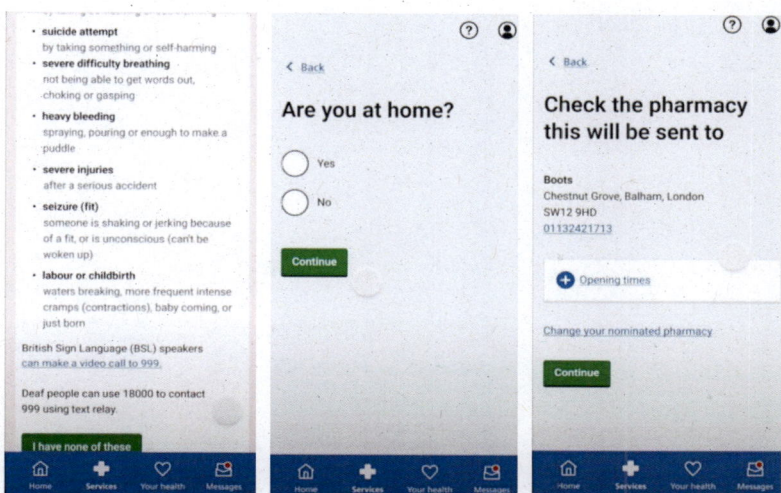

Figure 29. After checking the list of symptoms, the patient can select they have none of those.

Figure 30. The patient will be then asked whether they are home or not. At this stage, the patient can use 111 online.

Figure 31. To request a prescription, patients can click 'request repeat prescription' on the home page. The patient will be able to see and change their nominated pharmacy.

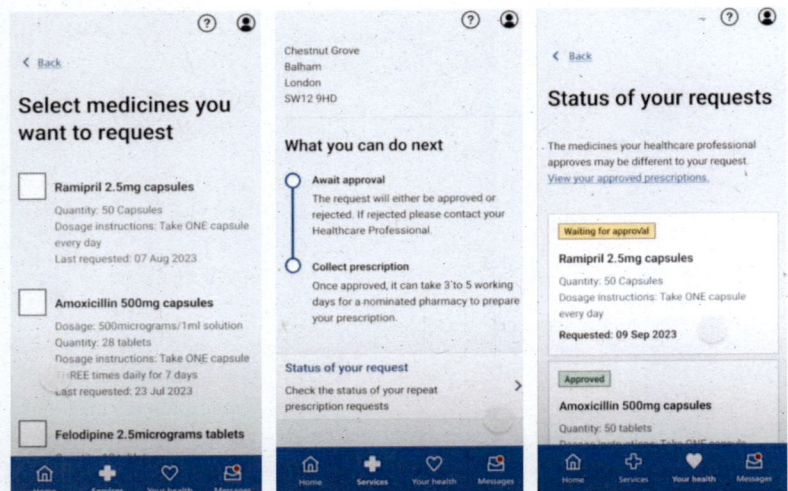

Figure 32. The patient will then see their medicines and select those needed.

Figure 33. Once the patient confirms, they can see what they can do next and check the request status.

Figure 34. The request status page shows whether a medicine has been approved or whether it is waiting for approval.

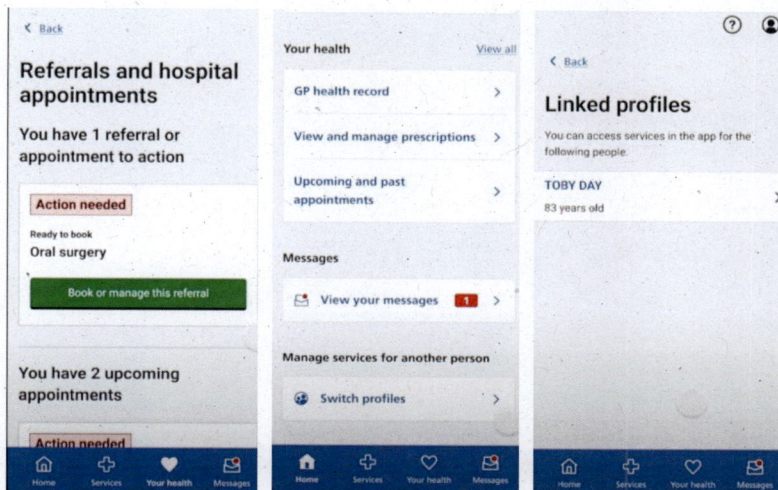

Figure 35. To view referrals and hospital appointments, patients can select 'upcoming and past appointments' on the App homepage and then 'hospital referrals and appointments.' Patients can book and manage the selected referrals.

Figure 36. From the homepage, a patient can navigate to the 'Switch profiles' section.

Figure 37. The patient will then see, upon receiving access from their GP, the linked profile.

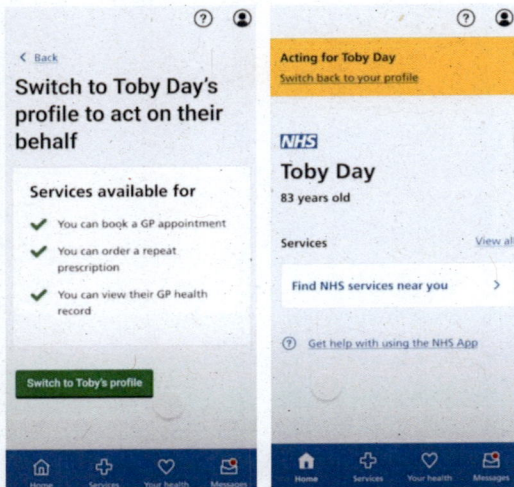

Figure 38. The next page shows which services the patient can use on behalf of the linked person.

Figure 39. While the patient is using the profile of the linked person, they can always use the yellow button at the top of the page to go back to their original profile.

The NHS App increasingly integrates informational resources, allowing patients to:

- Use NHS 111 online to answer questions and get instant advice or medical help nearby.
- Search trusted NHS information and advice on hundreds of conditions and treatments.
- Find NHS services near them.

Appointment booking

Suppliers include: DrDoctor, Netcall, Patients Know Best, Zesty.

Screenshots of Zesty inside the NHS app:

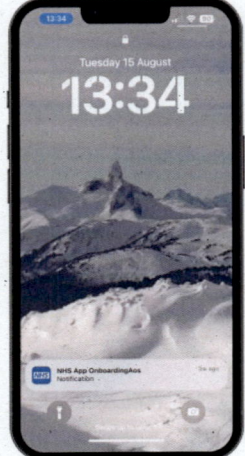 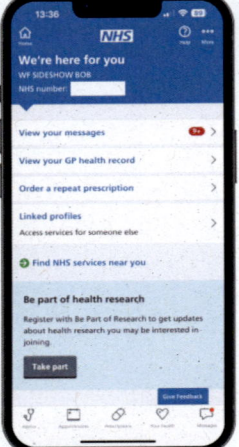 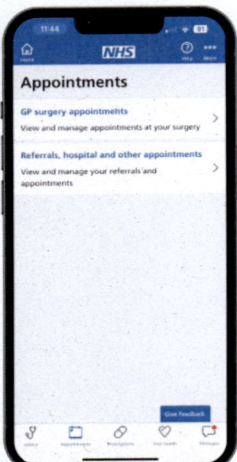

Figure 40. Patients will receive NHS App push notifications.

Figure 41. NHS App home page.

Figure 42. Patients can click on 'Appointments' on the menu at the bottom of the page. From the NHS App Appointments page, they can select 'GP surgery appointments' and 'Referrals, hospital, and other appointments.'

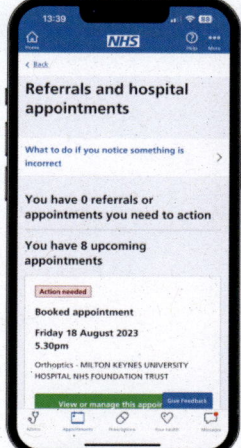
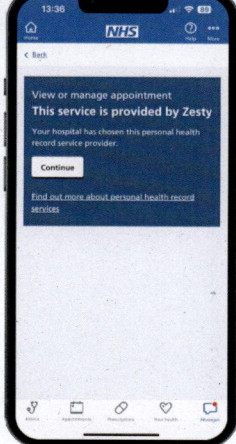
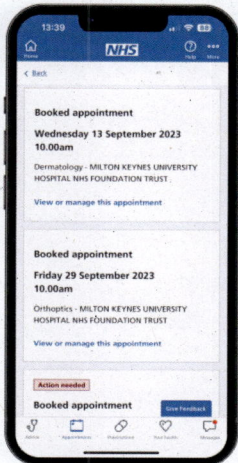

Figure 43. Once patients select 'Referrals, hospital, and other appointments,' they can see a list of referrals they need to action and their upcoming appointments. If patients want to view more details about an appointment or manage it, they can click on 'View or manage this appointment.'

Figure 44. The patients are then informed that this service is offered by Zesty.

Figure 45. Patients can see their booked appointments and whether any action is needed.

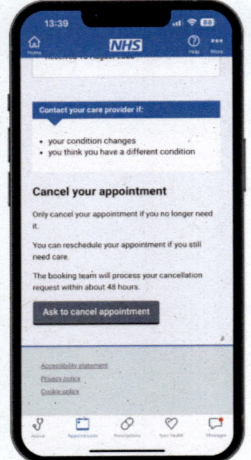
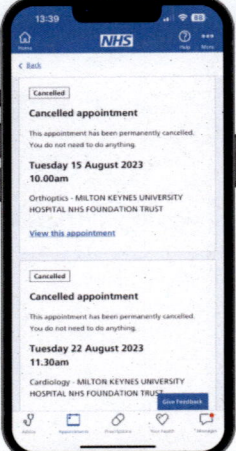
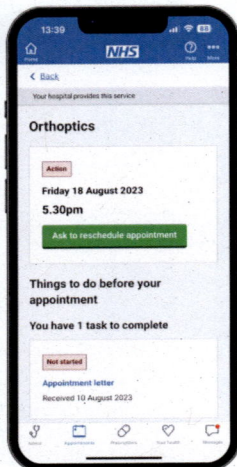

Figure 46. Patients can ask to cancel appointments through the App.

Figure 47. Cancelled appointments present a 'Cancelled' label.

Figure 48. Patients can also ask for appointments to be rescheduled.

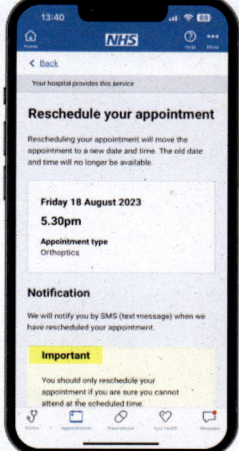
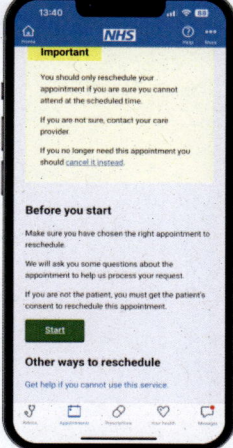
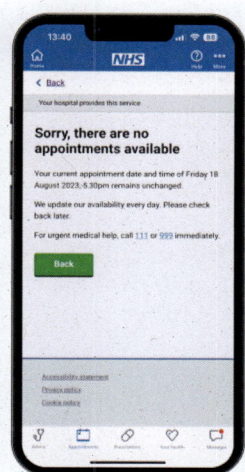

Figure 49. When asked to reschedule an appointment, the patients are presented with a page describing how the feature works and are warned that once the appointment is rescheduled, they can no longer attend at the old scheduled time.

Figure 50. Patients will read the full warning and then click on 'Start.'

Figure 51. If there are no other appointment slots available, patients will be shown the above screen.

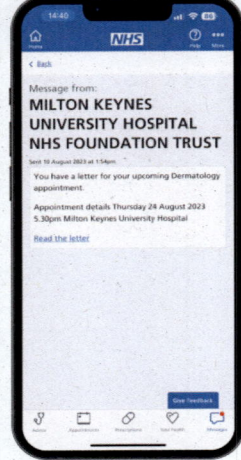
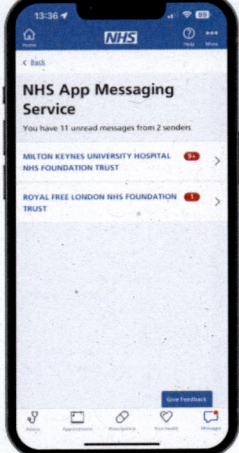
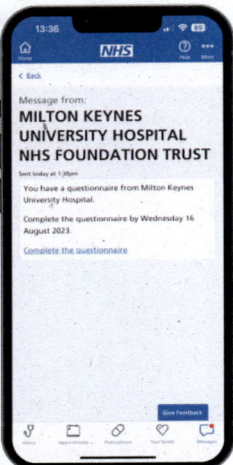

Figure 52. Patients can receive and access hospital letters, such as appointment letters, post clinic, and discharge summaries.

Figure 53. Patients can receive push messaging within the NHS App from multiple organisations.

Figure 54. Patients can receive and access pre-appointment, pre-assessment, or waiting list validation questionnaires.

Electronic consultations

Suppliers include: eConsult, accuRx, TPP (Airmid), engage health (mainly in primary care).

These apps allow patient-initiated triage, i.e., the patient answers the software's questions, so the software assesses and recommends urgency for clinicians.

Screenshots of eConsult inside the NHS app:

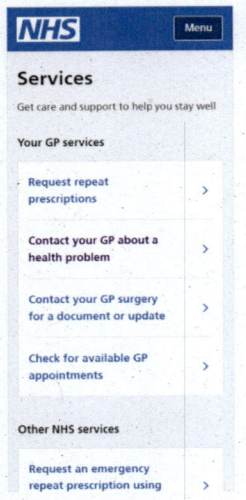

Figure 55. Services.

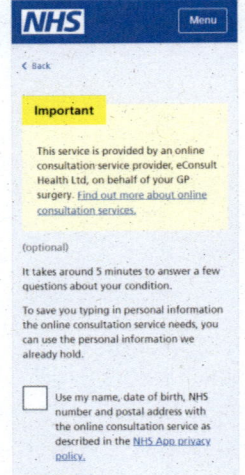

Figure 56. eConsult.

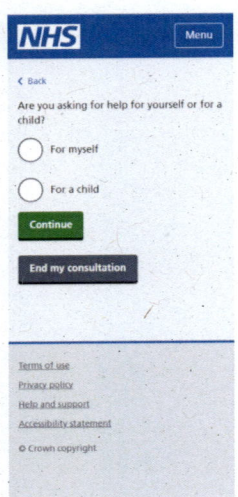

Figure 57. Child proxy.

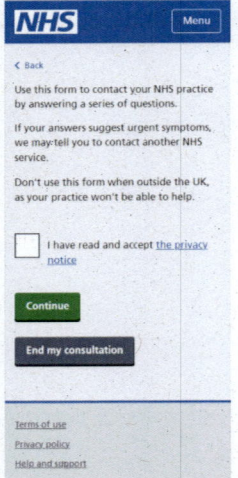

Figure 58. Privacy policy.

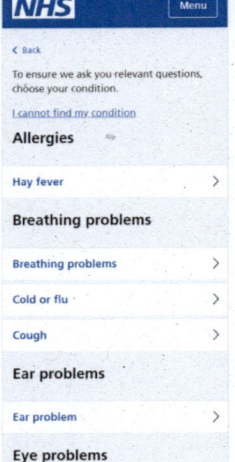

Figure 59. Condition list.

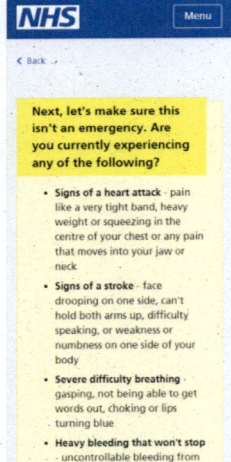

Figure 60. Safety netting.

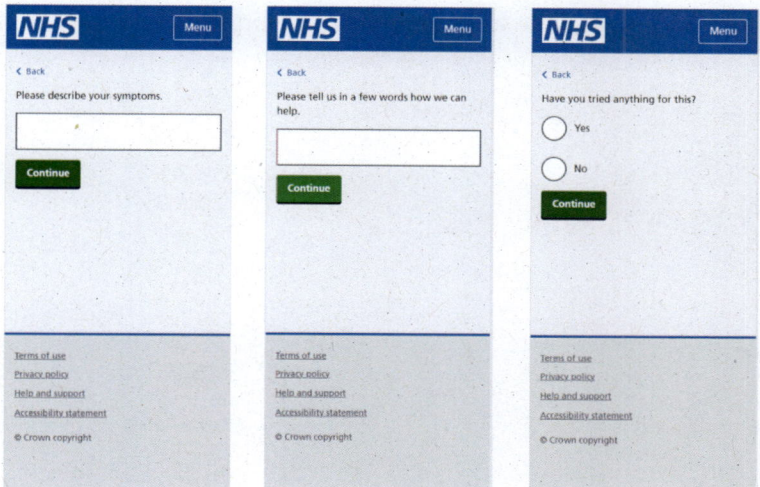

Figure 61. Describe symptoms.

Figure 62. How can we help?

Figure 63. Have you tried anything for this?

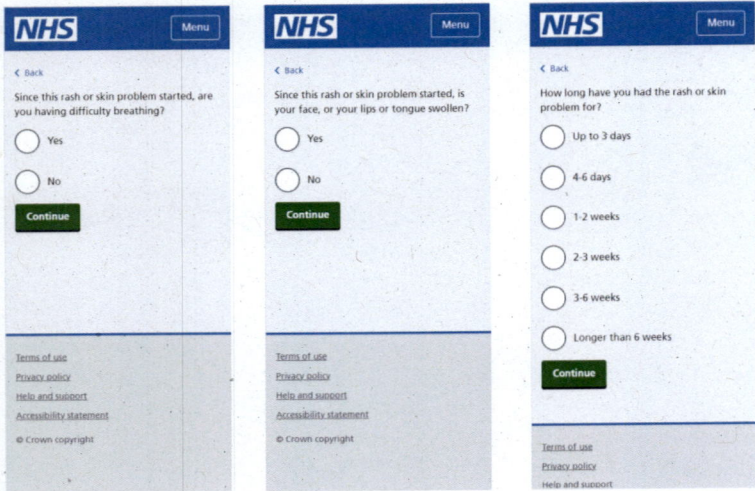

Figure 64. Clinical question.

Figure 65. Clinical question.

Figure 66. Clinical question.

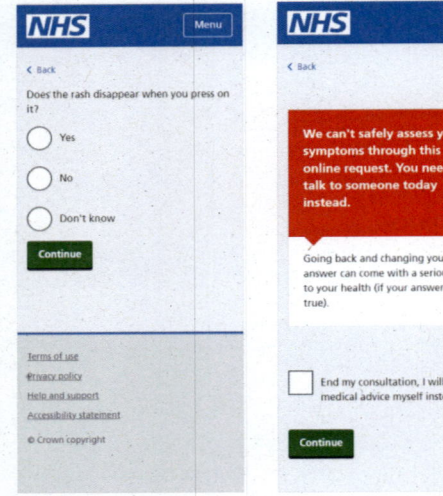

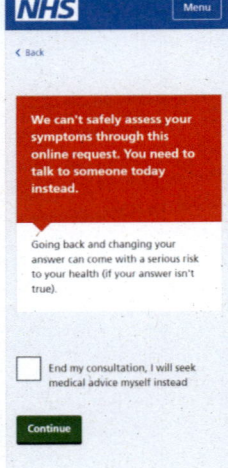

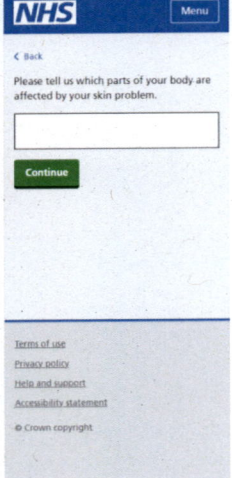

Figure 67. Clinical question.

Figure 68. Urgent symptom divert.

Figure 69. Clinical question.

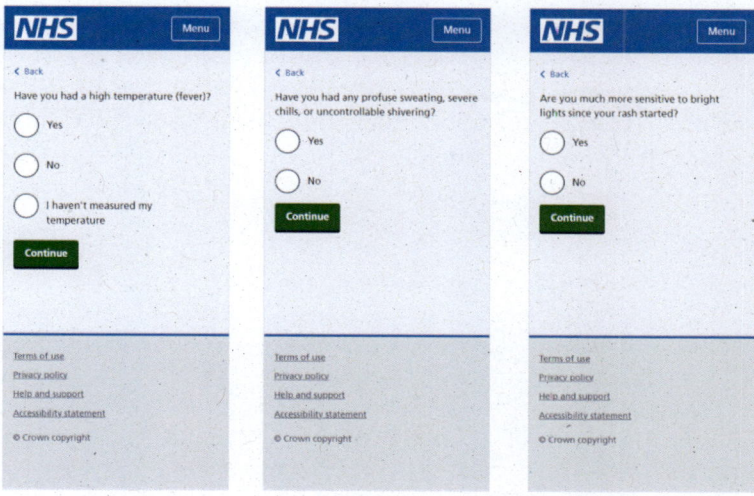

Figure 70. Clinical question.

Figure 71. Clinical question.

Figure 72. Clinical question.

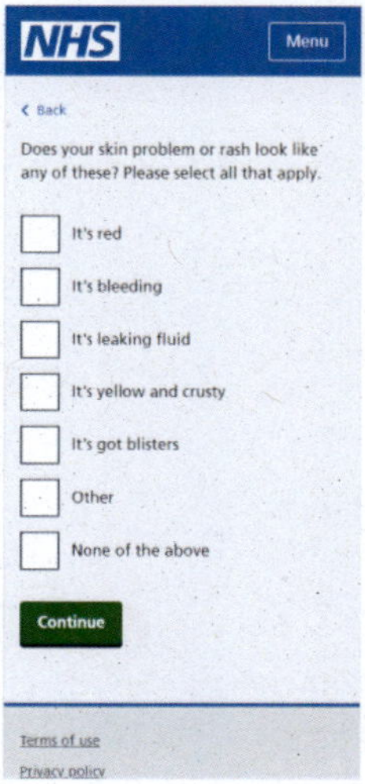

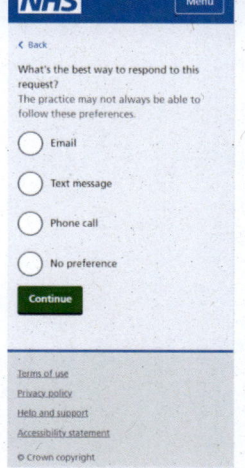

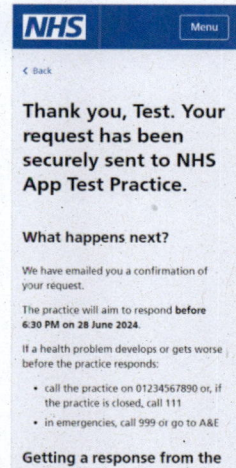

Figure 73. Clinical question.

Figure 74. Contact preferences.

Figure 75. Confirmation.

Personal health records

Patients Know Best (PKB) integrated with the NHS app in 2020. PKB gives the NHS App user full PKB functionality beyond the GP-only standard NHS App functionality.

Screenshots of Patients Know Best within the NHS app:

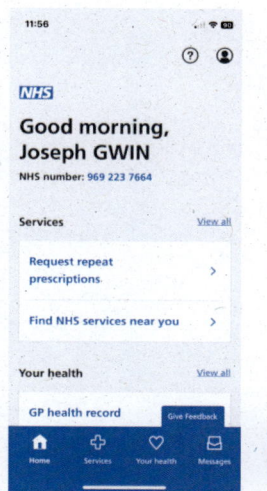
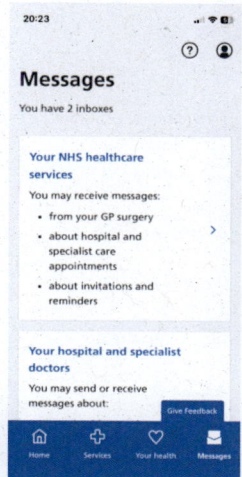
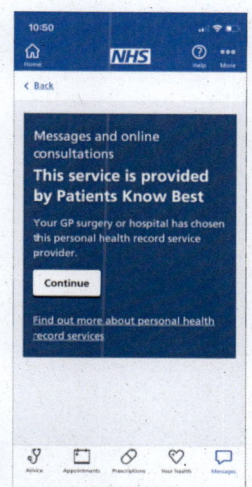

Figure 76. To view Messages, patients can click on 'View your messages' from the homepage or 'Messages' in the navigation menu.

Figure 77. They can then click on 'Your hospital and specialist doctors.'

Figure 78. Patients are informed that this service is provided by Patients Know Best. They can click 'Continue.'

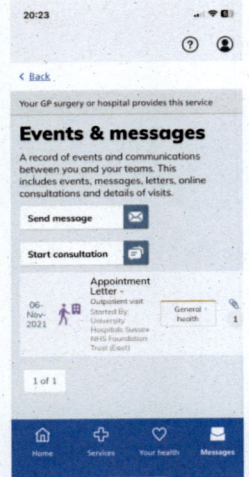

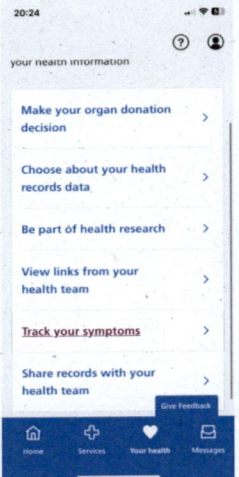

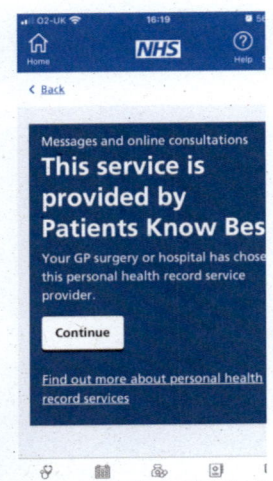

Figure 79. The Events & messages page displays letters and documents from integration engines and hybrid mail solutions. Includes free-text secure messages, with the option to attach photographs and videos.

Figure 80. To see the Library, patients can click on 'Your health' in the main NHS App navigation menu, then click on 'Your health choices' and 'View links from your health team.'

Figure 81. Patients are informed that this service is provided by Patients Know Best. They can click 'Continue.'

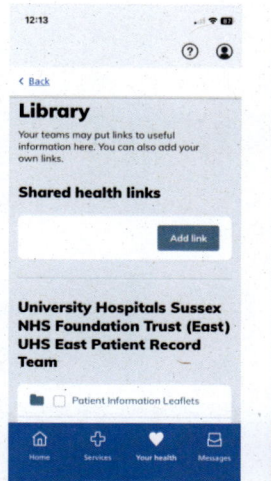

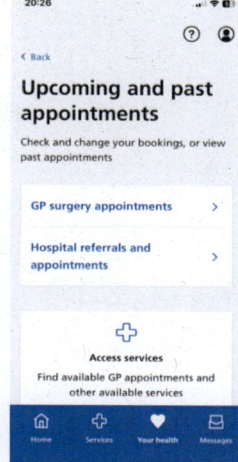

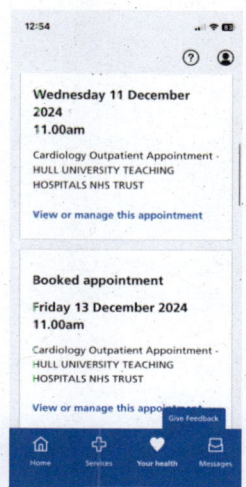

Figure 82. The Library contains links to external websites and documents from verified resources.

Figure 83. Patients can click on 'Upcoming & past appointments' from the NHS homepage or the 'Your Health' page. They can then click on Click on 'Hospital referrals and appointments' in the submenu and on 'Additional appointment information.'

Figure 84. Patients can see a list of their appointments and can click on 'View or manage this appointment' for any of them.

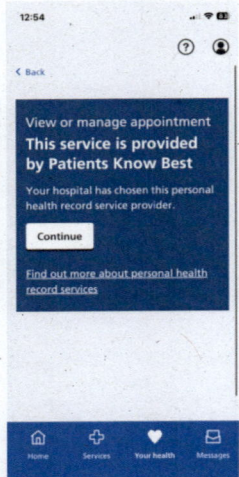

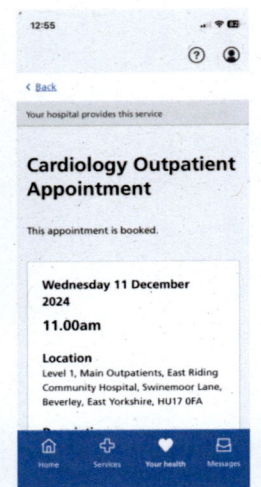

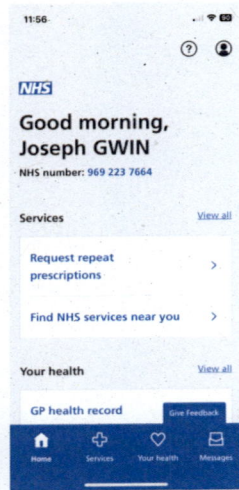

Figure 85. If the appointment is from PKB, patients will be directed to PKB. They can click 'Continue.'

Figure 86. The Appointments include data from EHRs, such as time, date, and location (and virtual consultation links). Patients can add other appointments they are aware of. Some organisations offer appointment messaging: this allows patients to send secure messages to reschedule or cancel their appointment.

Figure 87. To view their medications, patients can click on 'View and manage prescriptions' on the NHS App homepage or from the 'Your health' menu.

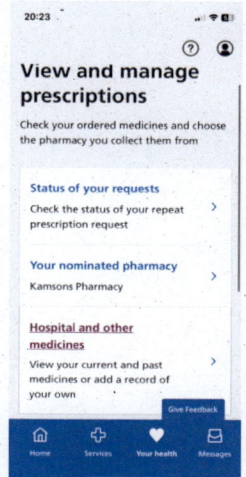

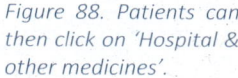

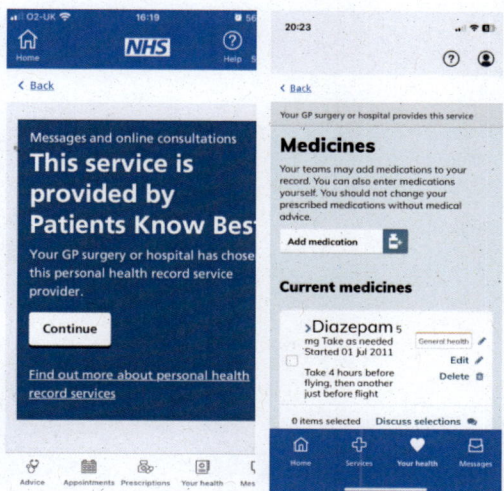

Figure 88. Patients can then click on 'Hospital & other medicines'.

Figure 89. Patients are informed that this service is provided by Patients Know Best. They can click 'Continue.'

Figure 90. Patients will land on the PKB Medicines page. Data can be entered by the patient, including over-the-counter substances, and can come from EHRs.

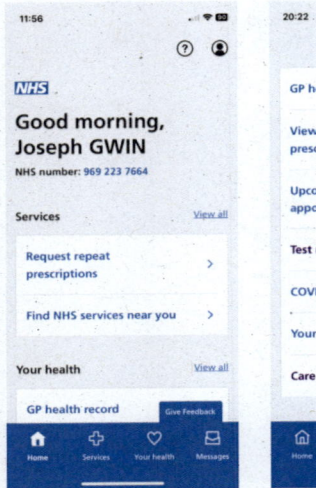

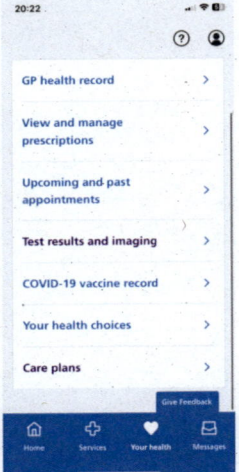

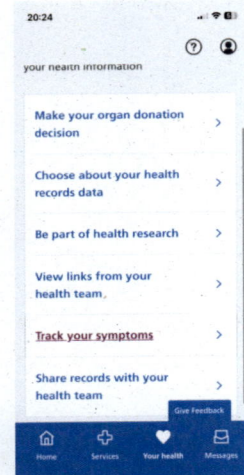

Figure 91. To view either Symptoms, Measurements, or the Journal, patients can click on 'Your health' in the main NHS App navigation menu.

Figure 92. They can then click on 'Your health choices.'

Figure 93. They can then click on 'Track your symptoms' and 'Track your health.'

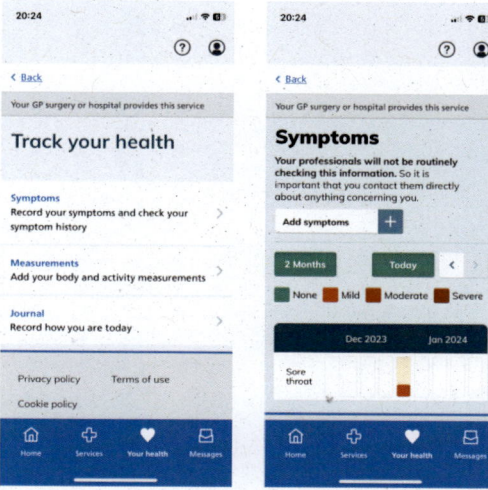

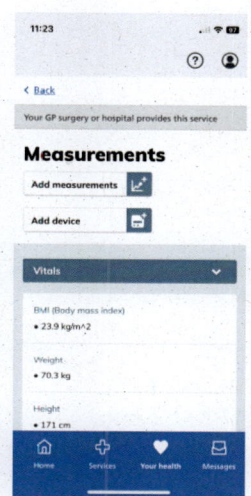

Figure 94. Patients can choose whether to see their Symptoms, Measurements, or the Journal.

Figure 95. On the Symptoms page, patients can add symptoms, including their severity.

Figure 96. On the Measurements page, patients can manually enter measurements. PKB also collects data automatically from OMRON, vital signs monitoring solutions, and other devices.

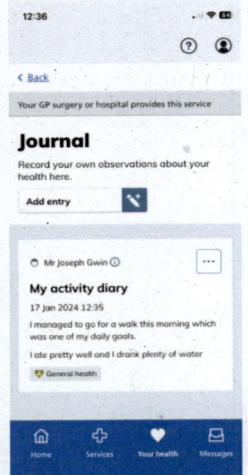
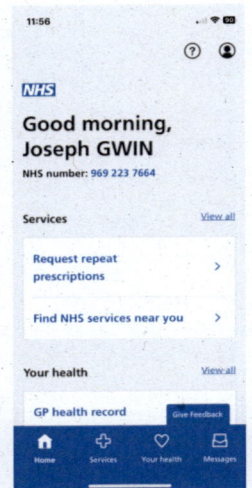
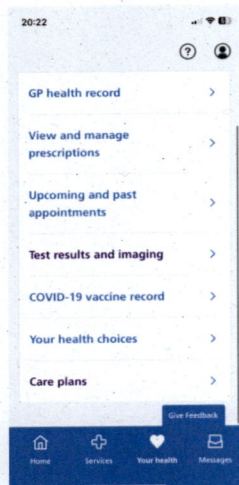

Figure 97. On the Journal page, patients can document what happened to them (thoughts and feelings) or questions to remember for their next appointment.

Figure 98. To view the Care plans, patients can click on 'Your health' from the main NHS App navigation menu.

Figure 99. Patients can then click on 'Care plans.'

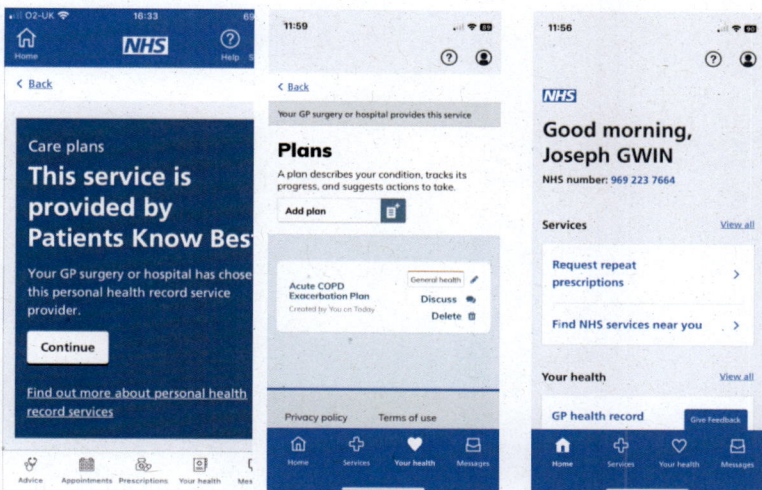

Figure 100. Patients are informed that this service is provided by Patients Know Best. They can click 'Continue.'

Figure 101. Care Plans can be co-edited and co-created by patients, professionals, and carers. They can include videos and interactive content, with patients contributing in their own words. They can display symptoms, test results, and measurements. They can feature action plans that share verified professional guidance.

Figure 102. To see imaging and test results, patients can click on 'Your health' in the main NHS App navigation menu.

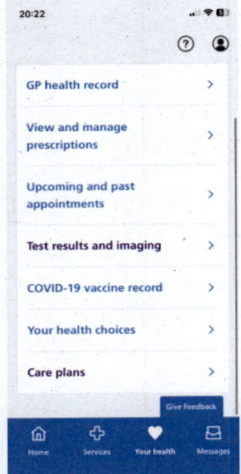

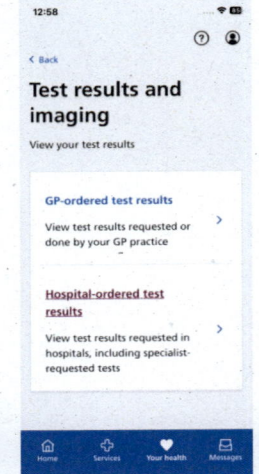

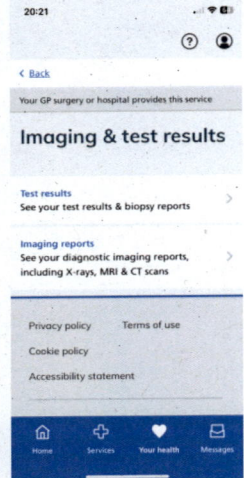

Figure 103. They can then click on 'Test results and imaging.'

Figure 104. Then click on 'Hospital-ordered Test results.'

Figure 105. They can then choose whether to see tests or imaging results.

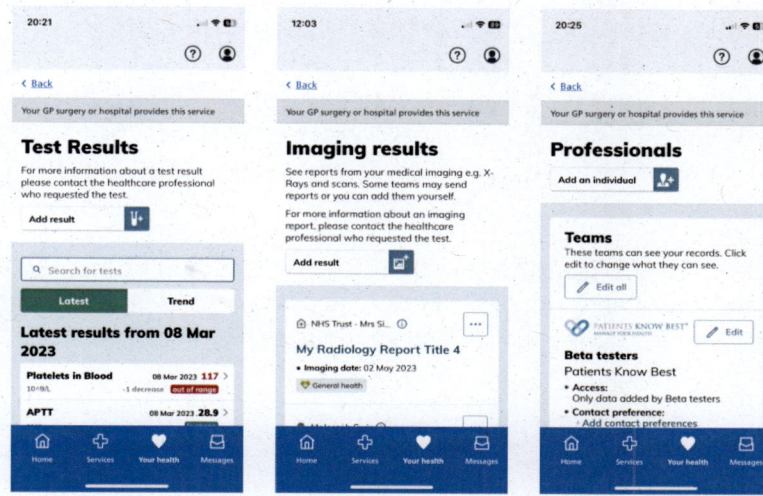

Figure 106. Test results have both charted and tabular displays, which include reference ranges and changes from previous results.

Figure 107. On the Imaging page, patients can view reports and associated images, including X-rays, MRI scans, and CT scans.

Figure 108. If patients click on "Your health" in the main NHS App navigation menu, then on 'Your health choices' and 'Share records with your health team,' they land on the Sharing page, where they can choose who can access their record and invite additional professionals to do so.

Challenges and areas for improvement

The main area for improvement is that the NHS App shows the features to patients based on the NHS organisation, not by the patient. So, either all the patients in a hospital can use a particular functionality or none.

Additionally, organisations must choose one supplier for each feature. For example, when it comes to appointment management, a hospital can only work with one appointment booking supplier for all appointments.

Statistics

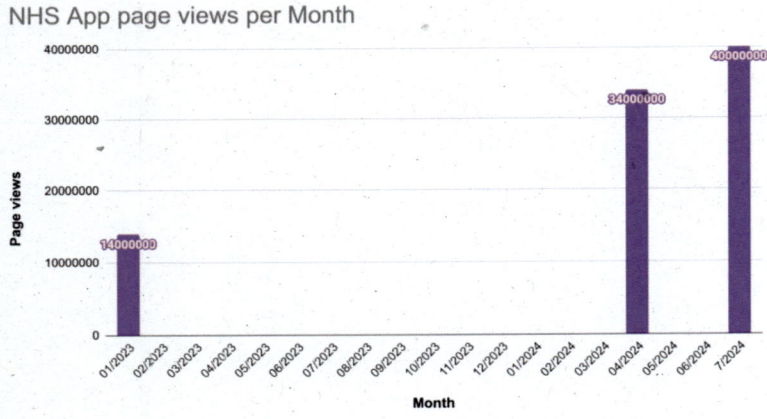

Figure 109. NHS App page views per month - from January 2023 to July 2024. No data is available for the empty months (PKB interviews, 2024).

April 2024

Based on PKB interviews:

- One in six users logs into the NHS App each month.

- A repeat prescription is processed every second, saving GPs an average of three minutes per interaction.
- 85% of GP records are accessible to patients. The remaining 15% are in breach of contractual obligations.
- In April 2023, 6 million patients accessed their GP records within a month. By April 2024, this number had increased to 17 million.
- The NHS 111 service via the app is nine times cheaper and four times faster than traditional phone calls.

December 2022

Older statistics showed cumulative sign-ups of over 30 million (Department of Health and Social Care et al., 2022). Over the year:

- 7 million new users registered.
- The app facilitated 1.7 million GP appointments and processed more than 22 million repeat prescriptions.
- GP records were viewed over 65 million times throughout the year.
- More than 21 million repeat prescriptions were ordered via the app, a significant increase from 9 million in 2021.
- Approximately 128,000 individuals registered their organ donation decisions through the app.
- New features allowed users to receive GP notifications and manage hospital appointments used over 800,000 times.
- Within four weeks of enabling the COVID-19 vaccine appointment feature, over 28,000 bookings were made through the app, representing 9% of all vaccine appointments.

Bibliography

- Al-Ubaydli, M., 2024. What makes the NHS app successful? Digital Health. Available at: https://www.digitalhealth.net/2024/07/what-makes-the-nhs-app-successful/ (accessed: 25 July 2024).

- Barclay, S., Lord Markham, C., Department of Health and Social Care, NHS Digital, NHS England, 2022. NHS App hits over 30 million sign-ups. Available at: https://www.gov.uk/government/news/nhs-app-hits-over-30-million-sign-ups (accessed: 12 October 2023).

- Department of Health and Social Care, NHS England, NHS Digital, The Rt Hon Steve Barclay MP, Lord Markham CBE. (31 December 2022). NHS App hits over 30 million sign-ups. Available at: https://www.gov.uk/government/news/nhs-app-hits-over-30-million-sign-ups (accessed: 12 October 2023).

- Duffy, D., 2020. Matthew Gould outlines the digital mission of NHSX. Hospital Times. Available at: https://hospitaltimes.co.uk/the-digital-mission-of-nhsx/ (accessed: 25 July 2024).

- European Observatory on Health Systems and Policies, 2022. United Kingdom: health system summary 2022. Available at: https://eurohealthobservatory.who.int/publications/i/united-kingdom-health-system-summary (accessed: 12 October 2023).

- Kc, S., Tewolde, S., Laverty, A. A., Costelloe, C., Papoutsi, C., Reidy, C., Gudgin, B., Shenton, C., Majeed, A., Powell, J. & Greaves, F., 2023. Uptake and adoption of the NHS App in England: an observational study. The British Journal of General Practice: The Journal of the Royal College of General Practitioners, 73(737), pp. e932–e940. Available at: https://pmc.ncbi.nlm.nih.gov/articles/PMC10562999/ (accessed: 3 November 2024).

- NHS app goes live with full rollout to GP practices promised by July. GP Online. Available at: https://www.gponline.com/nhs-app-goes-live-full-rollout-gp-practices-promised-july/article/1523685 (accessed: 25 July 2024).

- NHS, 2023. About the NHS App. Available at: https://www.nhs.uk/nhs-app/about-the-nhs-app/ (accessed: 12 October 2023).

- NHS Digital, 2024. NHS Digital Transformation: The Road Ahead (video). Available at: https://www.youtube.com/watch?v=90foL7lKn-Y (accessed: 25 July 2024).

- NHS Digital, 2024. The Future of NHS Technology (video). Available at: https://www.youtube.com/watch?v=Zpf3wnJvw20&t=28s (accessed: 25 July 2024).

- Preston, S., Keyfitz, N. and Schoen, R., 1972. Causes of death: life tables for national populations. New York: Seminar Press.

PATIENT PASSPORTS PROPOSAL FROM THE TIMES HEALTH COMMISSION FOR ENGLAND'S NHS

The proposal

On February 4th, 2024, after one year of research, the Times Health Commission presented a "report into the state of health and social care of Britain today" (Times 2024). It had a 10-point proposal for the NHS.

A ten-point plan for health

1 Create digital health accounts for patients, called patient passports, accessed through the NHS app, to book appointments, order prescriptions, view records, test results or referral letters and contact clinicians.

2 Tackle waiting lists by introducing a national programme of weekend high-intensity theatre lists to get through a week of planned operations in a day and create seven-day-a-week surgical hubs.

3 Reform the GP contract to focus on wider health outcomes, ensure prompt appointments and restore continuity of care. Encourage more super-practices and create community health centres.

4 Write off student loans for doctors, nurses and midwives who stay in the NHS. Debt should be cut by 30 per cent for those staying three years, 70 per cent for seven years and 100 per cent for ten.

5 Introduce no-blame compensation for medical errors with settlements determined according to need to ensure families get quick support and encourage the NHS to learn from mistakes.

6 A National Care System giving the right to appropriate support in a timely fashion. Equal but different from the NHS, it should be administered locally and delivered by a mixture of public and private sectors.

7 Guarantee that all children and young people requiring mental health support can get timely treatment and rapid follow-up appointments. Publish data on waiting times for all mental health services.

8 Tackle obesity by expanding the sugar tax, taxing salt, implementing a pre-watershed ban on junk food advertising and reducing cartoons on packaging to minimise children's exposure to unhealthy food.

9 Incentivise NHS staff to take part in research and put the case for research to their patients by giving 20 per cent of consultants and other senior clinicians 20 per cent protected time for research.

10 Establish a Healthy Lives Committee empowered by a legally binding commitment to increase healthy life expectancy by five years in a decade.

The first point of focus in the report addressed health data fragmentation and highlighted how technology can transform healthcare by improving efficiency and reducing costs. The solution found and proposed by the Commission is the creation of a 'Patient Passport,' according to which every patient treated by the NHS should have all their health information stored digitally in a single place, and every doctor who is treating a patient should be able to access that patient's record. As with a real travel passport, the Patient Passport should work seamlessly and be accessible and considered valid across any healthcare institution: GPs, NHS hospitals, pharmacies, and social care.

The Commission found that - as also highlighted in this research - there are similar systems already in place in other countries, such as Denmark and Estonia, while in the UK, within the NHS, there currently are around 40 to 60 types of electronic patient records, and 10% of hospitals do not have any and are still relying solely on paper.

Key points emphasized by the Commission include the importance of prioritizing prevention and allocating more resources towards it, placing patients at the forefront of their care, and empowering them to actively manage it.

In terms of the implementation methodology, the proposal is that the passport could be built upon and accessed through the NHS app - which would have to be improved accordingly to, among other things, include data from more healthcare providers.

Survey results

The Times also published data from YouGov polling for the commission:

- 81% of respondents support the patient passport proposal, with 10% against it.
- 89% of respondents believe that patients should have automatic access to their medical records.
- 56% of respondents think the benefits of being able to book appointments and access care online outweigh any potential privacy risk. 22% of respondents disagree with this.
- 68% of respondents would be happy for the NHS to allow other medical professionals to access their health records.
- 64% of respondents would be happy for their data to be used for research anonymously.

How does this map to a Personal Health Record and other similar concepts?

The report does not specify who should control access - the patient or the NHS providers. It does state that the patient should see everything. It also has an NHS-centric view of data sharing. So, while it has many of the properties of a PHR - a complete, accurate, real-time, persistent record that the patient can see for their own self-assessment and self-management, but also the provider access for safety and productivity - it leaves open the question of control and thus ownership.

NHS control means the NHS will miss out on non-NHS parties that can contribute to a citizen's care, including the patients themselves. As soon as the NHS "owns" such a passport, it also owns the risks: the clinical risk of seeing and acting on everything in the record to avoid liability, the technical risk of building such a platform, the security risk of managing access to so much data from so many sources.

The NHS does not want to take on such risks, according to our private interviews with NHS senior leaders. Government bureaucracies are also not able to take on such risks, as seen in other governments' IT projects. Thus, NHS ownership would not deliver the goals of the patient's passport, and we recommend an explicit commitment to patient ownership so that the patient's passport is a PHR.

As it was found in this research, many countries have attempted to leverage technology to digitise patients' records for the benefit of patients, professionals, and the whole healthcare system.

What is the Times Health Commission?

The Times Health Commission was formed in January 2023 to look into the future of health and social care in England. This came about due to various factors like the pandemic's effects, budget pressures, issues in A&E services, long waiting lists, health dispari-ties, obesity rates, and the aging population. The commission con-sisted of experts from different areas of health and social care.

To gather insights, the members visited medical facilities and care homes in the UK and abroad, including countries like Japan, Ireland, Israel, Denmark, and Spain. They wanted to learn from the best practices they observed before creating their 10-point plan.

Over 600 witnesses provided expert opinions, and the commission also conducted economic analyses, business surveys, opinion polls, and focus groups. These efforts aimed to get a comprehensive view of what's working well and what needs improvement (Sylvester, 2023).

Bibliography

- Digital Health.,n.d.Times Health Commission presents 10-point plan with digital at the top. Accessed at:https://www.digi-talhealth.net/2024/02/times-health-commission-presents-10-point-plan-with-digital-at-the-top/#:~:text=The%20Times%20Health%20Commis-sion%20was,issuing%20its%2010%2Dpoint%20plan. (accessed: 1 May 2024).

- Sylvester, R., Hayward, E., & Lambert, G., 4 February 2024. Pub-lic back 'patient passports' to share medical records with any doctor. The Times. Accessed at: https://thetimes.co.uk/arti-cle/nhs-data-shared-freely-times-health-commission-bqhrfwh83 (accessed: 4 February 2024).

- Sylvester, R., 15 January 2023. What is the Times Health Com-mission? Its aims explained. The Times. Accessed at: https://www.thetimes.co.uk/article/times-health-commission-explained-objective-commissioners-bvl2937gf?gad_source=1&gclid=CjwKCAjwkuqvBhAQEiwA65Xx QERSJk2nQgS-DWDRylo45QO9vi_67vC8mweo4kW2Cia4H-w-vX9R0xoC_JQQAvD_BwE (accessed: 4 February 2024).

ESTONIA

Estonia is Europe's biggest creator of billion-dollar tech companies per capita (Atomico, 2022). This private sector excellence started with the public sector investing in technology. Its post-independence government mandated computer programming for every child in school in 1997.

Country's healthcare system in a nutshell

Estonia's healthcare system provides universal coverage. The government is the payer and provider of most health care.

The Ministry of Social Affairs manages the Estonian Health Insurance Fund (EHIF). EHIF is funded through general taxation and is the primary buyer of healthcare services. The Ministry also coordinates national health activities such as professional certifications, pharmaceutical quality assurance, and public health initiatives.

Hospitals are mainly owned by the state, local governments, or public legal entities. Primary care centres, pharmacies, and outpatient clinics (unless affiliated with hospitals) are privately owned (World Health Organization, 2024).

92.9% of the population is covered by health insurance. This includes members of health insurance schemes and those with free access to state-provided healthcare services (Our World in Data, n.p.).

Public vs private

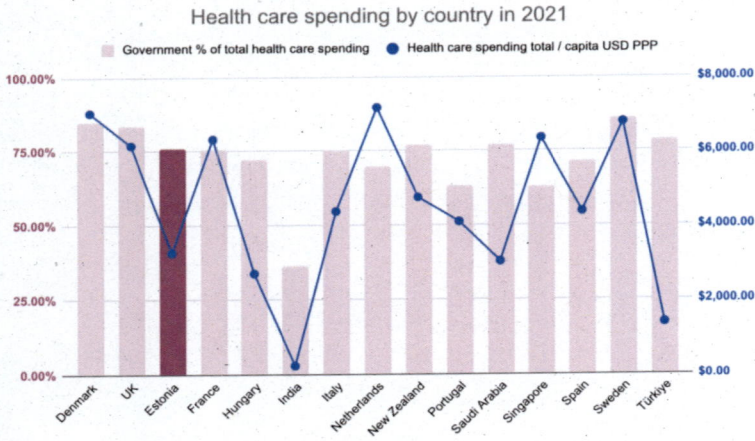

Figure 110. Source: The World Bank. The pink column refers to the public expenditure as a % of the country's total healthcare expenditure. The blue dot is the country's expenditure on health per capita, expressed in international dollars at purchasing power parity.

The national PHR

The e-health system in Estonia is called the 'Estonian Nationwide Health Information System' (EHIS). The Ministry of Social Affairs is responsible for it.

EHIS hosts central registers and databases, including those for hospitals, family doctors (general practitioners), pharmacies, school nurses, and medication interactions. It also hosts quality registers (such as cancer, HIV, and tuberculosis). It uses several nationwide registers, including the population and business registers.

The nationwide health information exchange platform is referred to as the nationwide Electronic Health Record (EHR) system. EHIS's EHR retrieves data to show in a standard format in the e-Patient portal, named Terviseportaal (Health Portal) (Metsallik et al., 2018). Data is from health care providers, who may be using different internal systems.

History

The evolution of the Estonian e-health system traces its roots back to the initial years of Estonia's independence and is linked to the efforts of its Prime Minister, Mr. Mart Laar, and his team. Mr. Laar held the position of Prime Minister in Estonia during two separate terms, from 1992-1994 and 1999-2002. During these periods, the strategic utilisation of information technology was perceived as key for advancing the country's economy. At that time, foundations were laid for numerous initiatives that now constitute the 'e-state' of Estonia, such as, apart from e-health, e-banking, e-documents, e-school, e-taxation, e-voting, and more.

There was a strategic emphasis on healthcare. Between 1990 and 2000, healthcare institutions embarked on developing proprietary information systems that incorporated electronic health records into their practices. At the same time, several small and medium-sized software companies dedicated to healthcare system development were founded. During this decade, discussions and conceptualisations for a nationwide e-health system began.

EHIS has been operating since 2008. The European Union contributed €1,196,200 and Estonia €398,735 to launch it (Metsallik et al., 2018). The eHealth Foundation was formed in 2005 to lead all digital health-based projects in Estonia (Willis, 2018).

Helmes, a private company, has managed the development of digital systems in Estonia for the past 15 years. The government's TEHIK (the Estonian Health and Welfare Information Systems Centre) selected Helmes. Helmes has played a key role in advancing the e-health sector, including the implementation of digital prescriptions, hospital information systems, and central patient administration. Their contributions cover other sectors, such as government, e-voting, e-justice, and security, to support the country's overall digital infrastructure (Helmes, n.d.).

What makes the Estonian system an exemplary e-government infrastructure is the seamless communication and data exchange among so many comprehensive services (Willis, 2018). Key contributors to the success of Estonia's e-health system include well-defined governance, legal clarity, a mature ecosystem, consensus on access rights, and the standardisation of medical data and rules for data exchange (Metsallik et al., 2018).

Architecture and features

EHIS has three layers: data, data transfer, and application—the data layer stores medical documents and images. The data transfer layer securely moves data over the internet between citizens and healthcare providers over the internet. The application layer delivers services and is in continuous development. It is tailored to the diverse needs of various stakeholders, including citizens, healthcare providers, government authorities, and policymakers.

EHIS is a federated system: healthcare-related software is independent and interconnected (Metsallik et al., 2018).

Main Elements of the Estonian Nationwide Health Information System (EHIS)

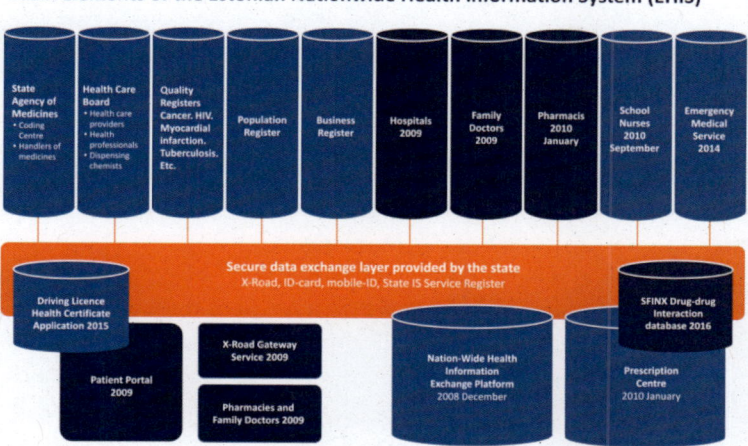

Figure 111. *Metsallik et al., 2018.*

The EHR centralises data retrieval from providers and standardises presentation on the e-Patient portal. Keyless Signature Infrastructure (KSI) Blockchain - a unique blockchain technology invented in Estonia - is used to ensure the integrity of retrieved electronic medical records as well as system access logs (e-Estonia).

The patient portal's users can:

- Log in using an ID card or mobile ID.
- See and update personal information and add contact details for close relatives.
- Access their medical data from healthcare providers.
- See referral letters and prescriptions.
- Authorise representatives for actions such as collecting e-prescriptions.
- Declare intention, e.g., organ donation.
- Access health insurance data.
- Hide sensitive information from doctors and representatives.

- Complete a health declaration form prior to an appointment.
- See a log of who has seen their data.

Challenges and areas for improvement

The development and implementation of the system faced several challenges (Metsallik et al., 2018)., including:

- **Resistance to Change**: Healthcare professionals were resistant, particularly in adopting a more standardised language for recording medical information in the e-health portal.
- **Reluctance to Share Data**: Some healthcare professionals were hesitant to share medical data with patients through the portal.
- **Data Quality**: Ensuring consistent and accurate data entry is a continuous challenge.
- **Semantic Interoperability**: Standardising medical terminology to achieve semantic interoperability of medical data is an ongoing effort.
- **Security and Authentication**: Ensuring robust security and electronic patient authentication is critical; blockchain technology has been instrumental in addressing this.
- **Privacy Concerns**: Users are concerned about potential secondary use of their data.
- **User Interface Development**: ensuring the usability and accessibility of the portal has been challenging and remains a priority.
- **Digital Skills**: A segment of the population lacks sufficient IT skills. To promote inclusivity, patients retain the option to keep accessing their data and services offline.

In terms of features, key areas for improvement include (PKB interview, 2024):

- Patient Data Entry: Patients currently cannot input their health data into the portal. The development team plans to enable this functionality in the near future.
- Device Integration: Patients are unable to connect personal health devices to their records.

Published outcomes - statistics

Every Estonian citizen who has visited a doctor at least once has an online e-Health record. 100% of Estonia's 1.3 million citizens have documents in the central database, 40 million documents in total. 100% of prescriptions issued are electronic. Since August 2022, the e-Prescription system has been interoperable with those in Finland, Portugal, Croatia, and Poland.

Doctors query EHIS 2.5 million times a month (e-Estonia, 2024).

Patient usage is high, demonstrating significant interest in accessing data. This supports the notion that providing patients with access to their health information empowers them and encourages a more active role in monitoring their health (Metsallik et al., 2018).

The use of digital health data in EHIS platform
December 2008 – May 2018

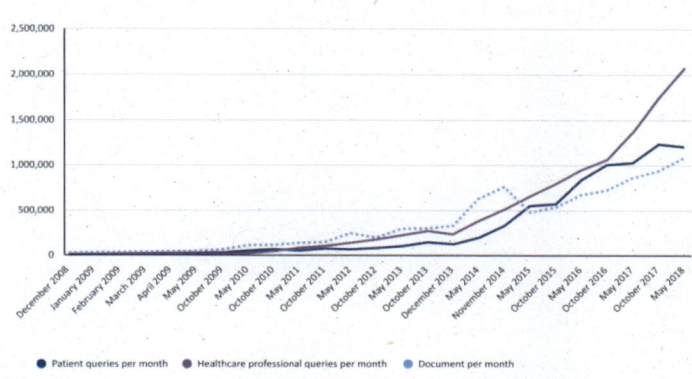

Figure 112. Metsallik et al., 2018.

Screenshots

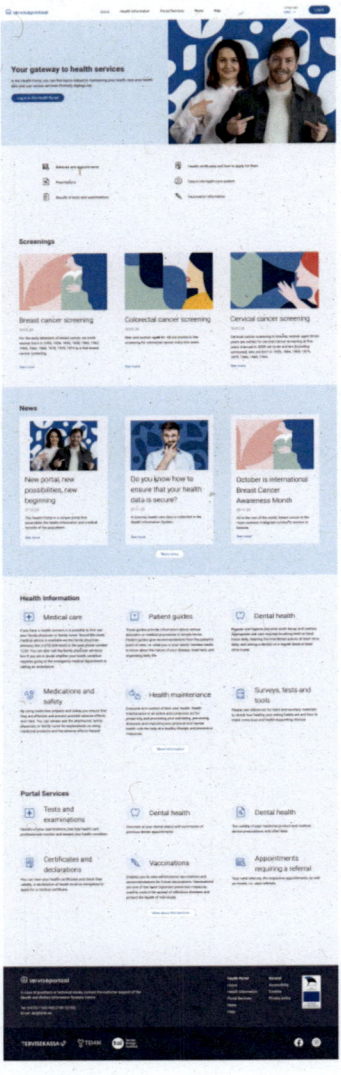

Figure 113. On the Terviseportaal homepage, patients can log in to access their records. The page outlines the purpose of the portal and the range of services. It also has valuable information about health maintenance, medication safety, screenings, and the latest health news.

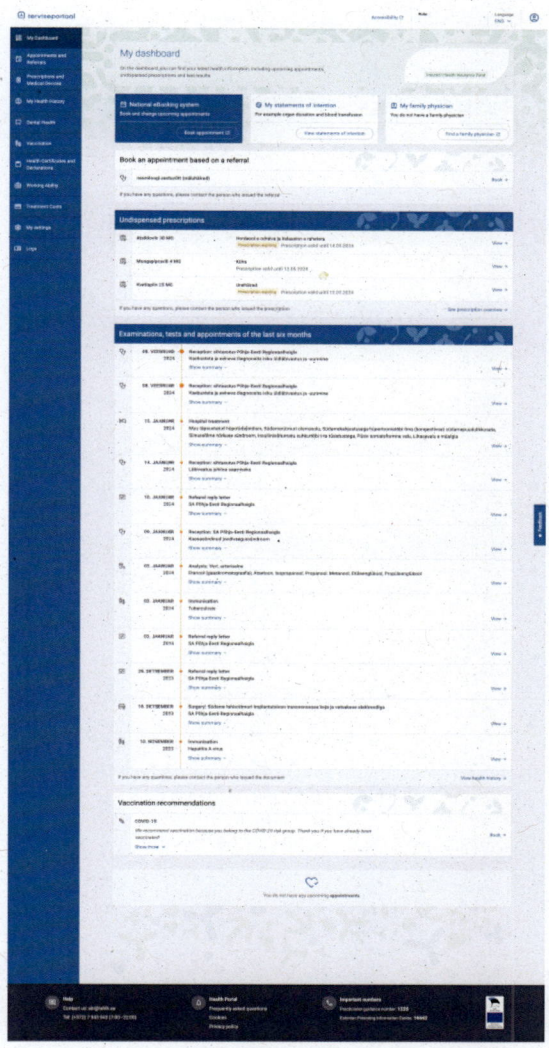

Figure 114. 'My Dashboard' is the portal's homepage. It links to the national appointment booking system and the statement of intention for organ donation and blood transfusion; patients can select a GP, book appointments based on referrals, and review prescriptions that have yet to be dispensed. Additionally, patients can view a six-month timeline of their examinations, tests, and appointments, along with a list of recommended vaccinations and details of any upcoming appointments.

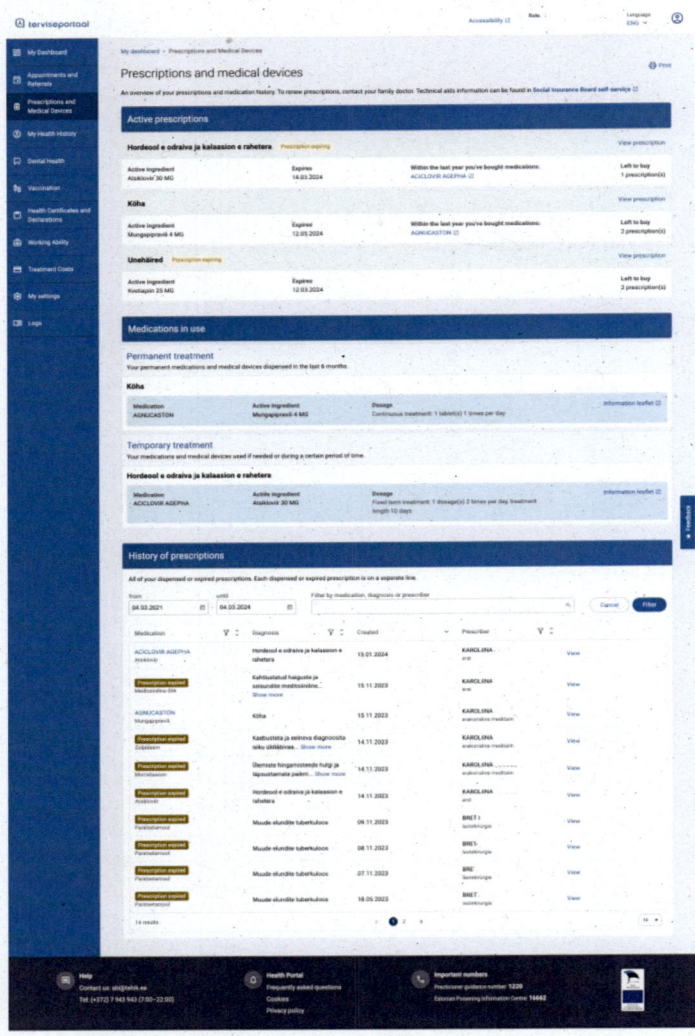

Figure 115. The 'Prescriptions' page provides an overview of both prescription and medication history. Active prescriptions include the names of medications, the expiration date of each prescription, and the quantity remaining to buy. Permanent medications and medical devices were dispensed in the last six months, and the name of the product, dosage, and information leaflet were detailed. The prescription history section includes a complete record of all dispensed medications and expired prescriptions, specifying the medication name, associated diagnosis, date of dispensation, and name of the prescriber.

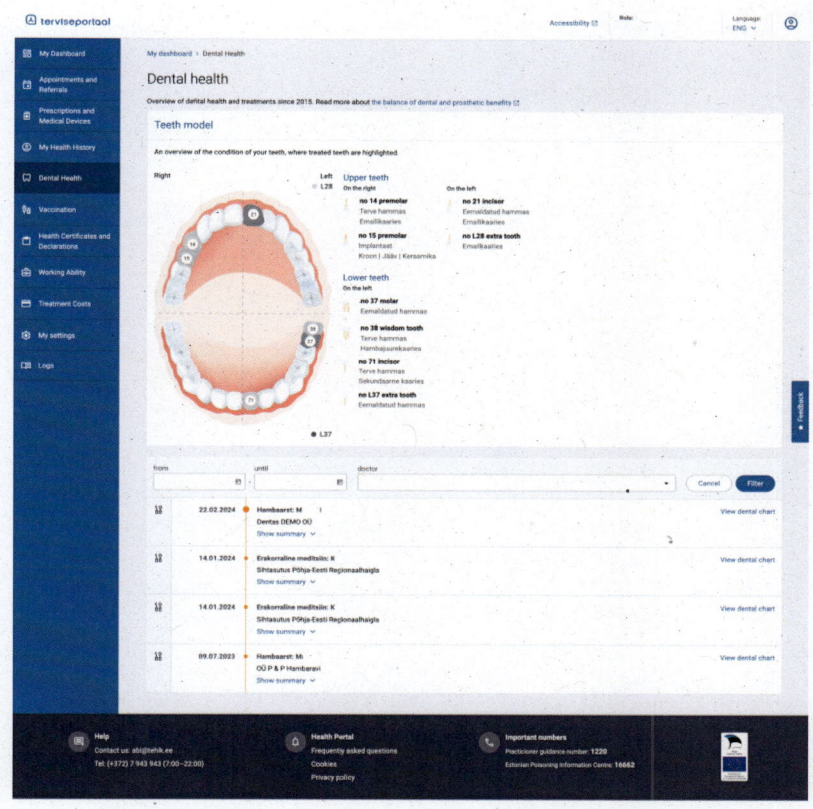

Figure 116. The 'Dental Health' section has an overview of their dental health and treatments dating back to 2015. This section features an image of a teeth model that visually represents the condition of their teeth, with treated teeth highlighted. Each highlighted tooth specifies the type of treatment received, such as implants or other dental procedures.

Bibliography

- Atomico, 2023. State of European Tech 23. Available at: https://stateofeuropeantech.com/ (accessed: 2 November 2024).

- e-Estonia, n.d. e-Health Records. Available at: https://e-estonia.com/solutions/healthcare/e-health-records/ (accessed: 16 July 2024).

- Helmes, n.d. Innovative platform improves the efficiency of the national population census. Available at: https://www.helmes.com/reference/innovative-platform-improves-efficiency-of-the-national-population-census/ (accessed: 16 July 2024).

- Lee, J., Park, Y.T., Park, Y.R. and Lee, J.H., 2021. Review of national-level personal health records in advanced countries. Healthcare Informatics Research, 27(2), pp.102-109. Available at: https://synapse.koreamed.org/articles/1146909 (accessed: 3 November 2024).

- Metsallik, J., Ross, P., Draheim, D. and Piho, G., 2018. Ten years of the e-health system in Estonia. In CEUR Workshop Proceedings, vol. 2336, pp. 6-15. Available at: https://ceur-ws.org/Vol-2336/MMHS2018_invited.pdf (accessed: 3 November 2024).

- Terviseportaal. Available at: https://www.digilugu.ee/login?locale=en (accessed: 11 July 2024).

- Willis, M., 2018. National digital infrastructures for healthcare: A comparative case of Estonian and British healthcare infrastructure. Centre for Technology and Global Affairs. Available at: https://ora.ox.ac.uk/objects/uuid:d6f98b44-8659-4ce2-8cab-b849f3bdb064 (accessed: 16 July 2024).

- World Health Organization, 2024. Estonia: health system summary 2024. Available at: https://eurohealthobservatory.who.int/countries/estonia (accessed: 25 July 2024).

- YouTube, 2019. Videopresentation: e-health. Available at: https://www.youtube.com/watch?v=gYzxzzQq2vg (accessed: 16 July 2024).

FRANCE

France's physicians are foundational to modern medicine. René Laennec invented the stethoscope in 1816. Jean-Martin Charcot joined Paris's Salpêtrière Hospital in 1862 and founded modern neurology, documenting multiple sclerosis and Parkinson's Disease. Louis Pasteur developed pasteurisation in 1864. Alexis Carrel trained with a seamstress to improve his surgical sewing, advancing vascular surgery and winning the Nobel Prize for Medicine in 1912.

Country's healthcare system in a nutshell

France's universal coverage operates under a statutory health insurance (SHI) model. SHI's wide coverage includes hospital care, physician services, long-term care, and prescription drugs. Patients are responsible for certain out-of-pocket expenses, such as coinsurance, copayments, and additional charges if fees exceed the covered amounts.

SHI funding is primarily from payroll taxes paid by both employers and employees, along with a national income tax and levies on specific industries and products. To offset out-of-pocket costs, 95% of French citizens also hold voluntary complementary private health insurance (VHI). It helps cover expenses for services like dental, hearing, and vision care.

Governance is shared between SHI funds and the national government. Recent reforms delegated some authority to regional health agencies. The central government retains considerable control over the system's overall management (World Health Organization, 2024).

99.9% of the population in France is covered: those who are members of health insurance schemes and those who have free access
to state-provided healthcare services (Our World in Data, n.p.).

Public vs private

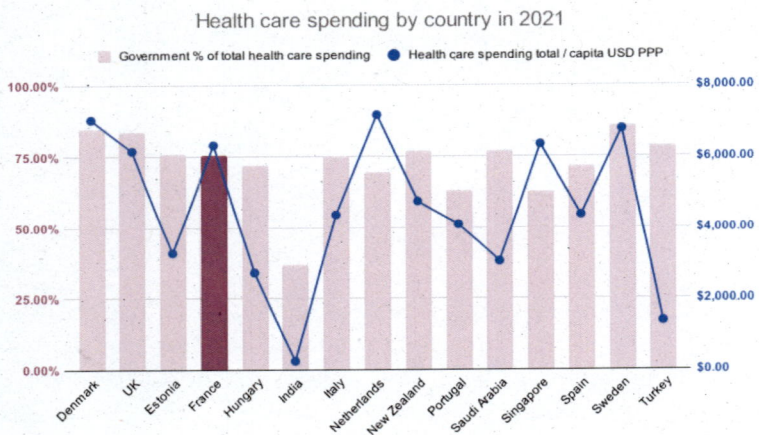

Figure 117. Source: The World Bank. The pink column refers to the public expenditure as a % of the country's total healthcare expenditure. The blue dot is the country's expenditure on health per capita, expressed in international dollars at purchasing power parity.

The national PHR

History

The "Ma Santé 2022" programme of the French Minister of Solidarity and Health set out a plan in 2019. Point 15 aimed to establish a
Digital Health Space to enable citizens to choose and access digital
health services securely and easily within the healthcare system.
Action 16 focused on providing healthcare professionals with a se-

cure platform for delivering clinical telemedicine services. And Action 8 mandated that all health professionals' software interoperate with the Digital Health Space by July 2023 (Simon and Moulin, 2022).

"Mon Espace Santé" (My Health Space) was the new name in a 2021 decree. The decree specified content and functionality (Simon and Moulin, 2022). The launch on January 1st, 2022, represented a milestone in the digitisation of healthcare services in France. The platform is available for all individuals under the umbrella of Health Insurance, with provisions for opt-outs (Simon and Moulin, 2022).

Mon Espace Santé is a partnership between the French government, a consortium led by Atos, and the National Health Insurance Fund (CNAM). Atos was awarded the project in November 2020, and the scope of their work included design, development, hosting, operation, and maintenance, all within a tight 13-month timeframe.

The consortium led by Atos comprises three notable French entities: Maincare Solutions, experts in Identity Management and health directories; Gravitee, an API platform specialist that contributes to the integration of diverse systems and functionalities; and Beezim, responsible for the platform's communication features (Atos International, 2022).

Features

Mon Espace Santé Data Sources and Services

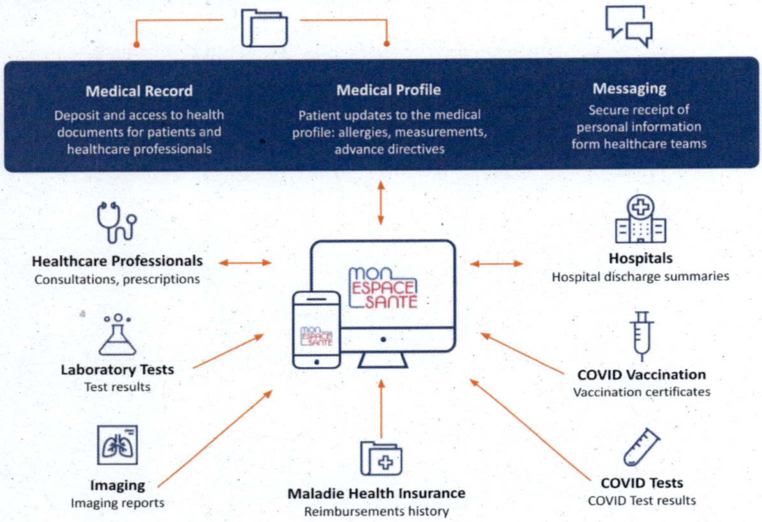

Figure 118. Ameli.fr

Patients using Mon Espace Santé can view and add to their health records. The platform's core feature, Mon histoire de santé (My Health History), tracks all patient interactions with the healthcare system, including visits to GPs, specialists, and pharmacies.

Other key sections of the record include (Mon Espace Santé, n.p.):

- **Medical conditions**: A summary of diagnoses.
- **Treatments and medications**: Details of current and past treatments.
- **Hospitalisation and disabilities**: Information on inpatient stays and any disabilities.
- **Risk factors**: Documentation of allergies, family medical history, and lifestyle factors.
- **Vaccinations**: Records of immunisations.

- **Health measures**: Metrics like weight, height, BMI, heart rate, and blood pressure.
- **Documents**: A section where both healthcare professionals and patients can upload important documents like vaccination certificates. Test results are also stored here, although patients must download the test report itself, as it is not displayed directly within the record.

Additionally, a **secure messaging** feature allows patients and healthcare professionals to communicate. Only the professional can start communication.

Patients can also share a summary of their profile with selected healthcare professionals. For families, Mon Espace Santé allows parents to activate profiles for their children, automatically linking these to the parent's records.

The **privacy control** feature lets a patient review all reports and decide which healthcare providers can access their information.

Challenges and areas for improvement

Challenges include (PKB interviews, 2024):

- Automatic data integration from hospitals remains inconsistent due to the platform being in its early stages, resulting in patient profiles often displaying only a partial view of their health data.
- Some information is not fully structured or coded. For instance, test results are typically provided as PDF files sent by healthcare facilities rather than being integrated into a structured format within the platform.
- As the statistics below indicate, the platform has not yet achieved widespread adoption.
- Patients are unable to view or manage appointments directly through the platform.

Published outcomes - statistics

An article published on 17 February 2023 by Agence du Numérique en Santé highlights the achievements of Mon espace santé in its first year. Since its launch, 65.7 million French citizens—representing over 90% of the insured population— have a profile. Of these, however, only 7.9 million (11.5%) have actively engaged with the platform.

From 1 January 2022 to January 2023, over 42.5 million health documents were shared with patients via Mon espace santé, and healthcare professionals have sent more than 1.7 million messages to users through the platform (Agence du Numérique en Santé, 2023).

As of 21 March 2024, 11 million patients (16.7%) and 45,000 general practitioners are actively using MES (L'Express, 2024).

Screenshots

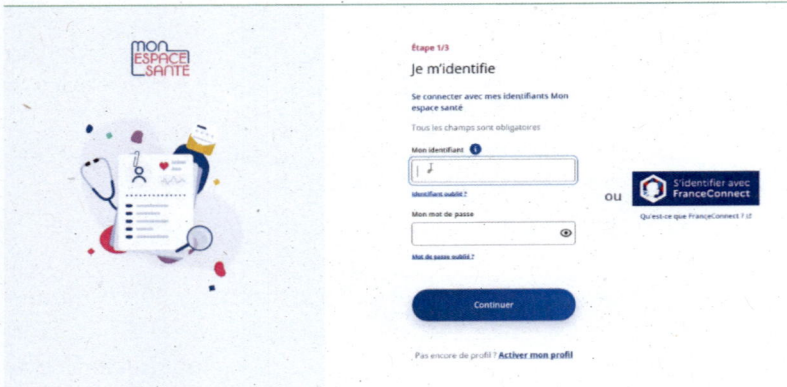

Figure 119. Login screen.

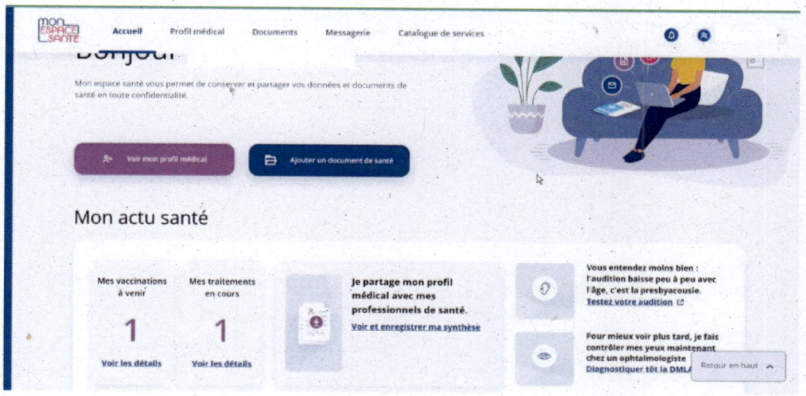

Figure 120. The Home page's buttons show patients their medical profile and allow them to upload health documents. The page also links to booked vaccinations and current treatments.

When a patient clicks to see their medical profile, they get this menu to navigate the record:

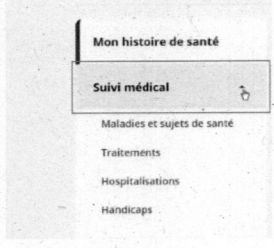

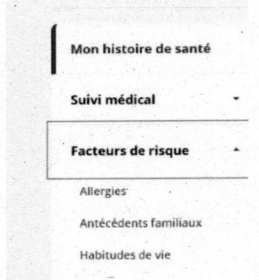

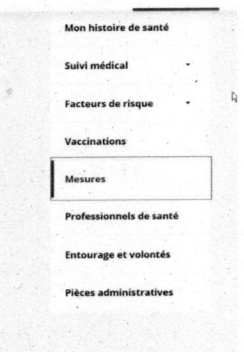

Figure 121. Within 'Suivi médical', there are various subtabs: patient's conditions, treatments, hospitalisations, and handicaps.

Figure 122. Within 'Facteurs de risque,' Risk factors, there are these subtabs: allergies, family history, and habits.

Figure 123. In the menu, patients can also access important sections, including vaccinations, measurements, healthcare professionals, and wills. The Wills section contains written wishes regarding the conditions for continuing, limiting, stopping, or refusing treatment or medical procedures in situations where the patient is unable to communicate, particularly in end-of-life scenarios.

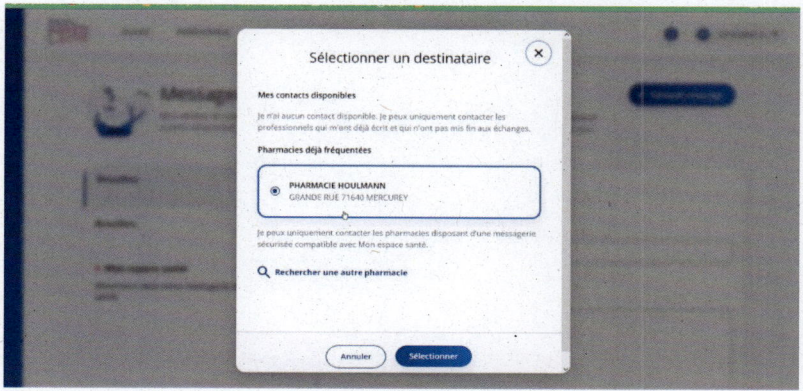

Figure 124. When patients click to select recipients for messages, they can only pick professionals who have previously communicated with them. However, patients can initiate an exchange with pharmacies.

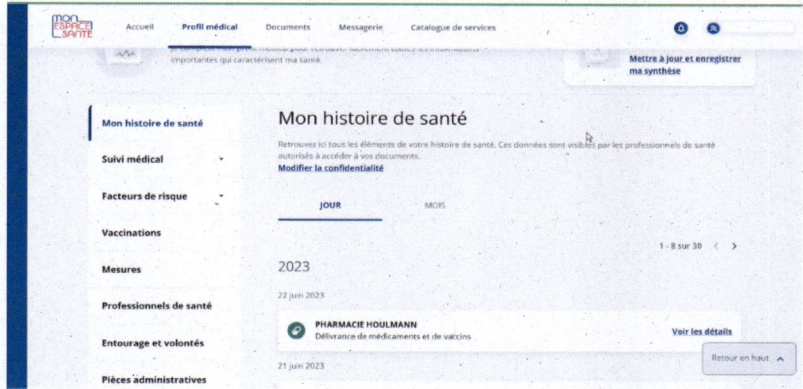

Figure 125. The My Medical History section provides an overview of the patient's healthcare journey. This includes records of consultations with healthcare professionals and any interaction with healthcare providers. Patients can click on an event to see more information about it.

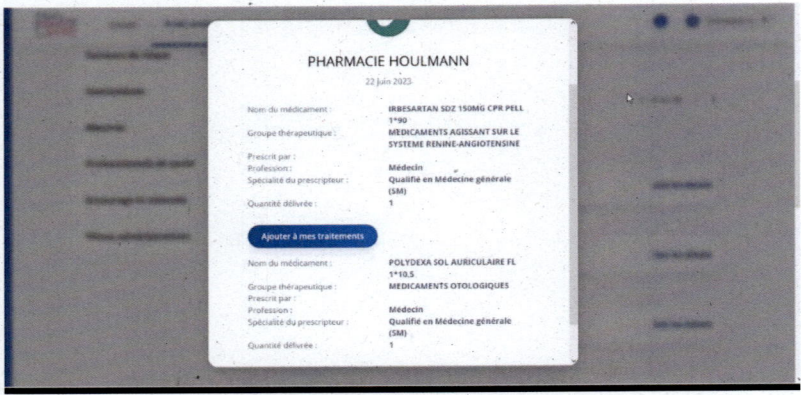

Figure 126. When patients click on the event from the previous screen, they can view detailed information about their transactions. In this case, the event was the patient buying a prescribed medication. This detailed view includes specifics about the medication purchased, the pharmacy where the transaction took place, and the type of doctor who prescribed it - in this instance, a general practitioner.

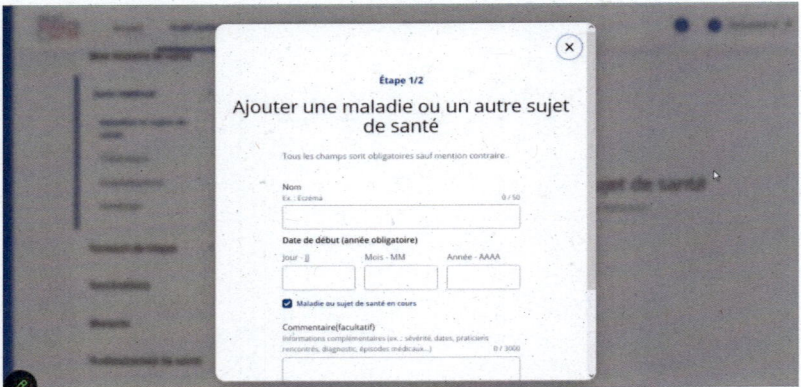

Figure 127. Patients can add a condition to their record by typing its name directly into the designated field. They are also required to specify the date the condition first appeared and can include any supplementary information that may be relevant.

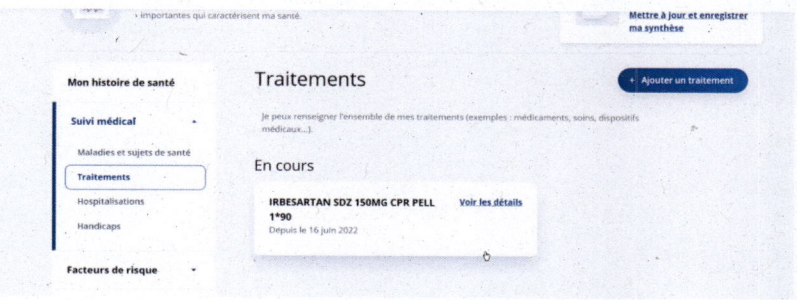

Figure 128. In the Medications section, patients can view information about the medications they are currently taking. They also have the option to add a new medication.

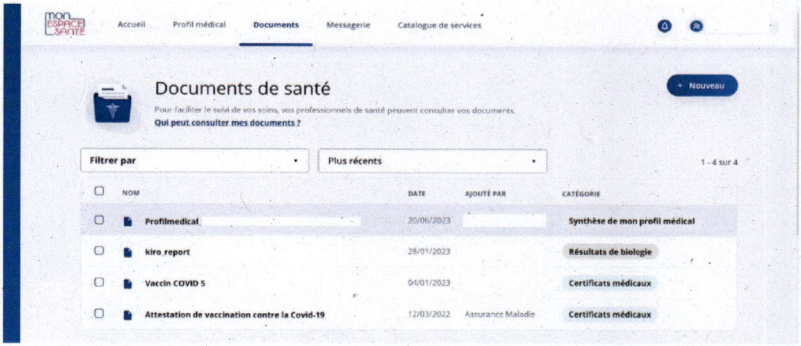

Figure 129. In the Health Documents section, patients can access important documents, including PDFs of test results (which are not coded within the platform) and COVID-19 vaccine certificates, among others. While some healthcare providers automatically upload information to this section, this is not always guaranteed, as the platform is still relatively new.

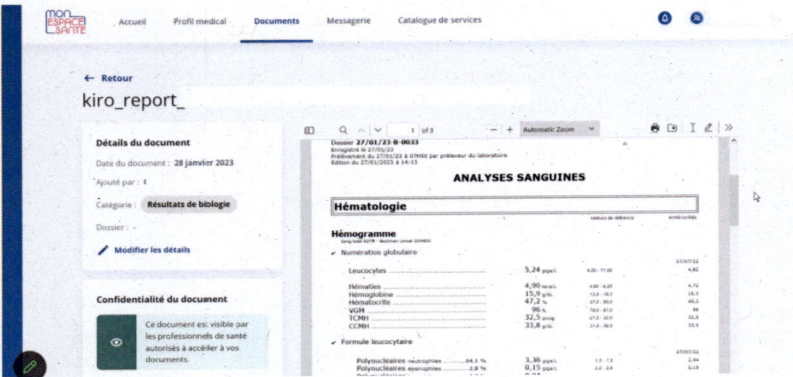

Figure 130. When patients open the test results in the Documents section, they are presented with a PDF view of their results.

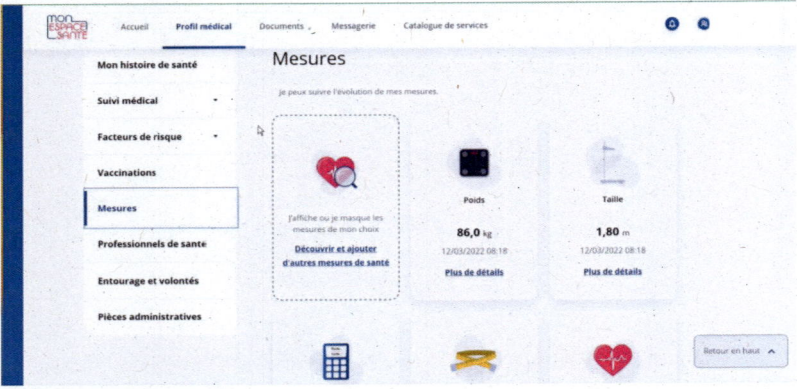

Figure 131. In the Measurements section, there is a dedicated tab for each type of measurement. Patients have the option to add these measurements manually or have them recorded by healthcare professionals. Currently, there are no integrations available with hospital systems or devices, and the data is not coded or structured. This section includes various measurements, such as weight, height, and more (see next screenshot).

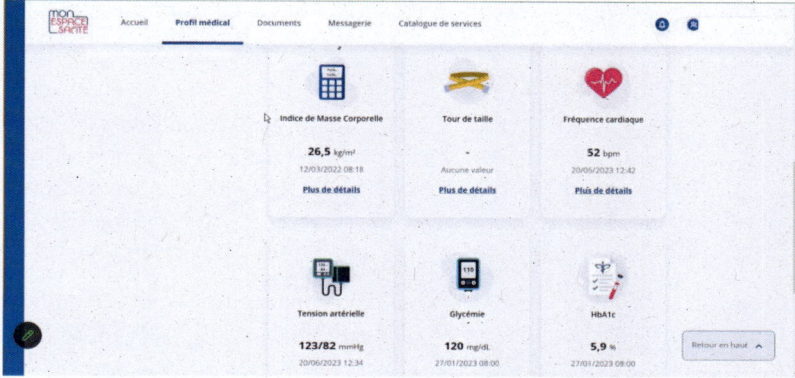

Figure 132. Other measurements include body mass index, waist size, heart rate, blood pressure, blood glucose, and hemoglobin A1C (HbA1C).

Bibliography

- Agence du Numérique en Santé, 2023. Mon espace santé a 1 an! Available at: https://esante.gouv.fr/actualites/mon-espace-sante-1 (accessed: 18 November 2024).

- Atos International, 2022. Atos successfully deploys Mon Espace Santé, France's online health platform. Yahoo! Finance. Available at: https://finance.yahoo.com/news/atos-successfully-deploys-mon-espace-091000705.html?guce_referrer=aHR0cHM6Ly93d3cuZ29vZ2xlLmNvbS8&guce_referrer_sig=AQAAADikyhlgsw7wl8s3ZW_OBJsmDRWARPuuGjHtoZwUYmM-B7rlV06bwH4tb4dZ9ozlzoIP7V4iT1T3awlB0wY4q1Sgr-_e1JtwlyXO6e39Yb8pm4lf7wRCbQay6q0AIsTW1Ku8_3sYdyC75nrsgjv6chVlk7mhLiA79P6hWJ1c3yiN&guccounter=2 (accessed: 30 October 2023).

- Fischer, A., 2024. "Mon Espace Santé", une action de santé publique bienvenue. L'Express, 21 March. Available at: https://www.lexpress.fr/sciences-sante/mon-espace-sante-une-action-de-sante-publique-bienvenue-par-le-pr-alain-fischer-MALU573CHVAXBJ7AZNRKQVBRSI/ (accessed: 20 April 2024).

- Mon Espace Santé.,n.p. Public service to manage your health. Accessed at: https://www.monespacesante.fr/ (accessed: 30 August 2023).

- Simon, P. and Moulin, T., 2022. Téléconsultation, télé-expertise, télésurveillance médicale: l'apport de «Mon Espace Santé». Bulletin de l'Académie Nationale de Médecine, 206(5), pp.643-647. Available at: https://www.sciencedirect.com/science/article/pii/S000140792200111X (accessed: 3 November 2024).

- The Commonwealth Fund, 2020. France: International Health Policy Center. (online) Available at: https://www.commonwealthfund.org/international-health-policy-center/countries/france (accessed: 18 July 2024).

- World Health Organization, 2024. France: Health System Summary 2024. Health System Summary. 20 May 2024. (online) Available at: https://eurohealthobservatory.who.int/countries/france (accessed: 25 July 2024).

HUNGARY

Hungarians' inventiveness may begin with their language. The language has a complex grammar style that trains cognitive agility. Due to migration and then isolation, the language is unrelated to most surrounding European neighbours. The small nation's speakers have to learn a different language structure to communicate with the rest of the world, further training cognitive agility. John von Neumann (creator of computing architecture), Charles Simonyi (creator of Microsoft Office), and Andrew Grove (co-founder of Intel) are all Hungarian-American technologists.

Country's healthcare system in a nutshell

Hungary's single health insurance covers nearly all residents. Its range of services is more limited compared to other European Union countries.

Since 2011, reforms have centralised the system, with the national government overseeing strategic direction, financing, regulations, and most specialist and inpatient care. The Ministry of Human Capacities manages the system through the National Healthcare Service Centre (ÁEEK), which coordinates care, plans hospitals, and oversees licensing. In 2012, the central government took control of local hospitals from county and municipal authorities, with ÁEEK managing these state-owned facilities.

The single health insurance fund is administered by the National Institute of Health Insurance Fund Management (NEAK), which is supervised by the Ministry of Human Capacities. Funding is derived from payroll contributions and government transfers.

Healthcare delivery is predominantly hospital-based, with the national government directly managing hospitals and providing most inpatient and outpatient services, though some local governments still operate polyclinics (World Health Organization, 2023).

Health insurance covers the entire population of Hungary, including both members of health insurance schemes and those with free access to state-provided healthcare services (Our World in Data, n.p.).

Public vs private

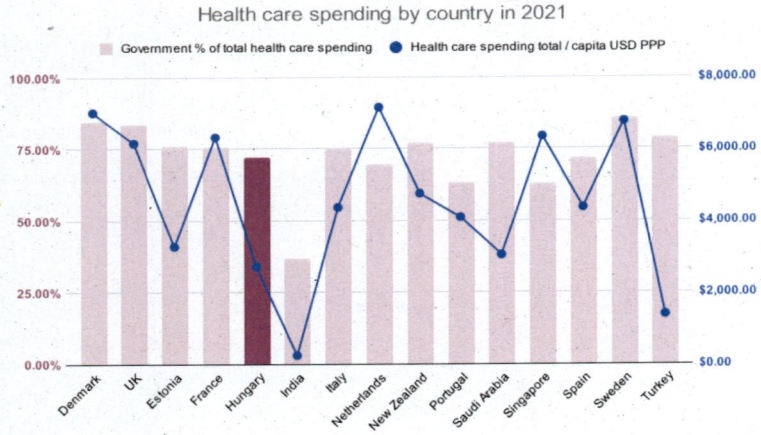

Figure 133. Source: The World Bank. The pink column refers to the public expenditure as a % of the country's total healthcare expenditure. The blue dot is the country's expenditure on health per capita, expressed in international dollars at purchasing power parity.

The national PHR

History

The National eHealth Infrastructure and its specialised modules were established under the Social Infrastructure Operating Programme. Funding was from the European Union and the Hungarian State. Total investment amounted to 4.87 billion Hungarian forints (approximately 13.15 million USD). Continuous development of the system is ensured through close cooperation between the Hungarian State and the European Union. For example, project no. 1.9.6 of the Human Resource Development Operating Programme focused on establishing the Electronic Health Service and Data Integration System (EESZT).

EESZT interconnects previously fragmented healthcare data systems across the country and collects all data into a central system. This enables treatment locations to access the necessary information seamlessly. Another key objective was to provide modern centralised services, such as electronic prescriptions, electronic referrals, and medical documents, as well as the eProfile. These promote the widespread adoption of modern healthcare practices.

EESZT usage has been mandatory since November 2017 for publicly funded healthcare providers and pharmacies. Non-publicly funded providers (including private practitioners) must provide data to the central implant and prosthesis registries and for the National Ambulance Service since November 2018. Since June 2020, private providers with valid operating licences performing outpatient medical or dental activities have also been required to report data to the EESZT (EESZT, n.d.-a; EESZT, n.d.-b).

Historical patient data has not yet been incorporated, so only data entered after joining the system is visible.

EESZT's History

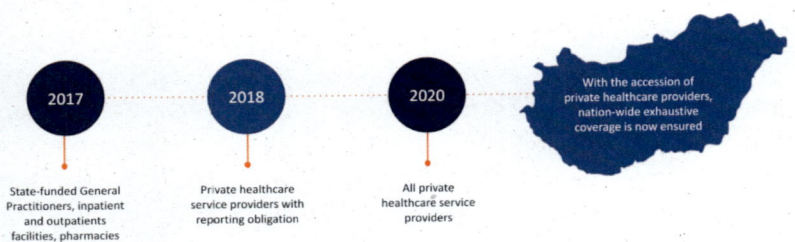

| 2017 | 2018 | 2020 | With the accession of private healthcare providers, nation-wide exhaustive coverage is now ensured |

State-funded General Practitioners, inpatient and outpatients facilities, pharmacies

Private healthcare service providers with reporting obligation

All private healthcare service providers

Figure 134. Source: History of EESZT - EESZT Információs portál

Features

Most hospitals in Hungary are integrated with EESZT. This integration ensures that data added locally to a hospital's electronic health record (EHR) is automatically uploaded to EESZT. Authorised health professionals—such as hospital staff, general practitioners, and pharmacists—can access data from EESZT through their organisation's systems. Access is role-based; for example, pharmacists can only view prescription information.

Patients can access their medical data through the EESZT citizen portal and mobile app. Features include seeing:

- **Prescriptions** and dispensed medications, including medical aids.
- **Referrals** for specialist consultations.
- **Health documents** such as outpatient **appointment reports and notes**, admission, and discharge documents.
- **COVID-related data**, including vaccination certificates, test results, and health certificates. Patients can also book COVID-19 vaccinations.
- **Test results**.

- **eProfile**, which includes critical health information such as allergies, pregnancy status, and implants. This profile contains health data rarely subject to change, uploaded by the GP, and could be life-saving if accessed during emergency care.

The Event Catalogue shows the patient a log of all healthcare service usage, whether in outpatient or inpatient facilities or at family doctor services.

Patients can also monitor who has accessed their data. They can customise settings to receive email notifications about specific EESZT events, controlling what data is displayed to physicians based on their permissions and preferences (EESZT, n.d.).

Challenges and areas for improvement

Key areas for improvement (PKB interviews, 2024) include:

- **Limited Patient Input Capabilities**: The platform currently allows patients to input limited types of health measurements. They are unable to manually add other essential medical data, such as allergies, detailed medical histories, or additional health documents (e.g., files or reports).
- **Lack of Direct Communication Between Patients and Professionals**: EESZT does not allow direct communication between patients and healthcare professionals. So, patients cannot use the platform to consult or follow up with doctors.
- **No Device Integration**: While patients can manually enter data measured by external health devices (e.g., wearable fitness trackers), there is no direct integration between these devices and the EESZT system.

Published outcomes - statistics

The latest statistics are from the 19th of April 2021 and are available at https://web.archive.org/web/20210419151255/https://e-egeszsegugy.gov.hu/web/eeszt-information-portal/the-role-of-the-eeszt-in-hungarian-healthcare.

"Today, more than 26 thousand health professionals and 13 thousand pharmacy staff use the system in Hungary. Starting from 2020, more than 22,000 institutions have access to the EESZT infrastructure, including private service providers."

This number breaks down as follows (EESZT Information portal, 2021):

- There are more than 6000 active general medical practitioners, as well as:
  - more than 300 outpatient institutions
  - more than 100 inpatient institutions
  - more than 3,000 pharmacies
  - more than 8,800 private healthcare institutions
- The details of more than 600 million receipts have been entered into the EESZT.
- An average of 800,000 new electronic prescriptions (ePrescription) are ordered daily.
- By June 2020, there was a 90% increase in the monthly prescription of electronic prescriptions.
- Annually, 75 million medical documents (e.g., medical records, outpatient data sheets, discharge summaries) and approximately 180 million doctor-patient appointments are recorded online in the EESZT system in Hungary. This amounts to a daily average of 300,000 medical documents recorded in the Infrastructure."

Screenshots

Screenshots are available on our website, phrs4govs.org.

Bibliography

- EESZT., n.d. The Role of the EESZT in Hungarian Healthcare. Available at: https://e-egeszsegugy.gov.hu/web/eeszt-information-portal/the-role-of-the-eeszt-in-hungarian-healthcare (accessed: 13 September 2023).

- EESZT., n.d. Citizen Portal - Main Page. Available at: https://www.eeszt.gov.hu/hu/nyito-oldal (accessed: 13 September 2023).

- EESZT., n.d. EESZT Information Portal - The History of EESZT. Available at: https://e-egeszsegugy.gov.hu/web/eeszt-information-portal/history-of-eeszt (accessed: 13 September 2023).

- World Health Organization, 2023. Hungary: Country Overview. (online) Available at: https://eurohealthobservatory.who.int/countries/hungary (accessed: 13 September 2023).

INDIA

The last time Indians were anyone's subjects [...]
was when the queen of England ruled India. And so,
to underscore the central importance of the indi-
vidual in data protection, the data subject is re-
ferred to, in India, as the data principal. Extending
this principle even further, the data controller is re-
ferred to as the data fiduciary since it holds the
data principal's personal data in trust.

Justice B.N. Srikrishna said this when the Indian government tasked him with drawing up a new regulatory framework for data protection. Changing the naming convention was one of his first acts (Rahul, 2023).

Country's healthcare system in a nutshell

The Indian Constitution mandates that the government ensure the "right to health" for all citizens, with each state responsible for providing free access to healthcare services (Tikkanen et al., 2020).

Statistics on health insurance coverage reveal a significant increase from 2010 to 2024. In 2010, only 12.5% of the population had health insurance (Our World in Data, n.p.). By 2017-18, this figure had risen to approximately 37% (Tikkanen et al., 2020). By 2021, the National Institution for Transforming India (NITI Aayog) reported that about 70% of the population was covered by some form of health insurance, including state government schemes, social insurance programmes, and private insurance (NITI Aayog, 2021).

Historically, the government introduced various health insurance schemes targeting specific groups, with coverage levels differing across states. However, despite these efforts, India's healthcare system has remained underfunded. This has resulted in critical shortages of healthcare infrastructure and workforce, lengthy wait times, and perceptions of poor quality in public health services. Consequently, the private sector has long played a dominant role in healthcare provision (Tikkanen et al., 2020).

Furthermore, the introduction of government health insurance schemes has not significantly reduced the burden of out-of-pocket expenses, leaving many patients to bear healthcare costs directly (Tikkanen et al., 2020).

The graphs below illustrate out-of-pocket expenditures in India from 2000 to 2024 and the change in the percentage of the population covered by health insurance from 2010 to 2024.

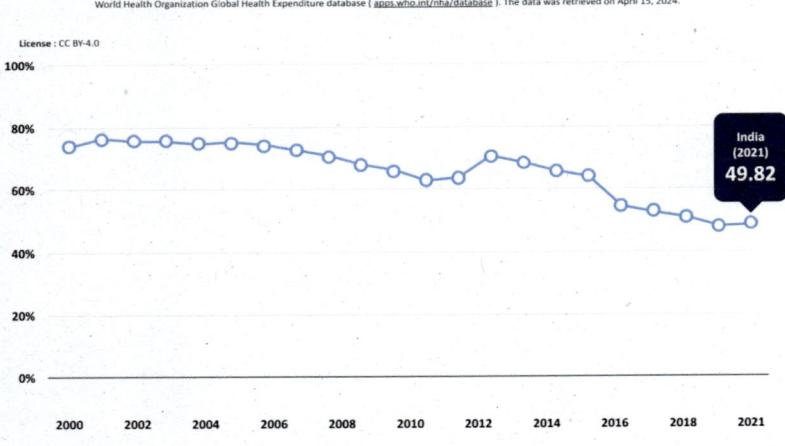

Figure 135. Source: World Bank, 2024.

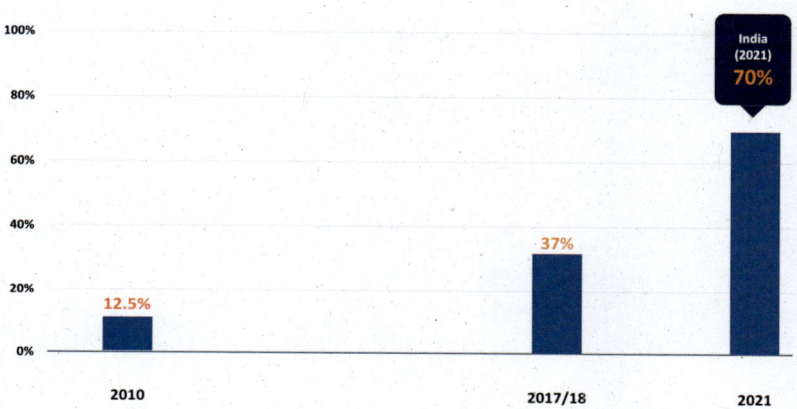

Figure 136. Source: Our World in Data; Tikkanen et al., 2020; NITI Aayog, 2021.

Public vs private

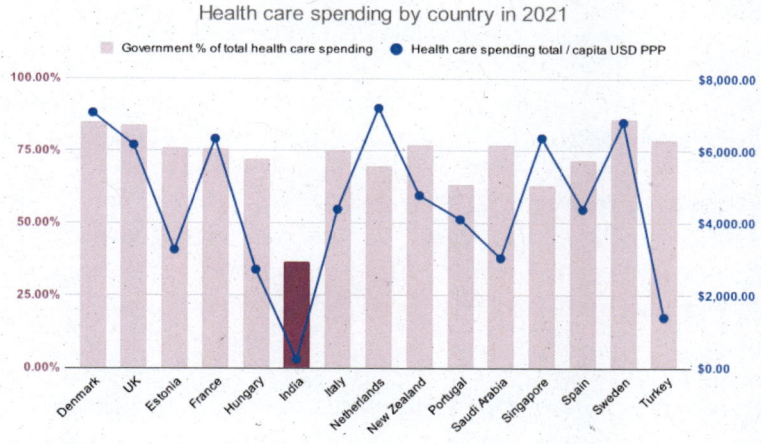

Figure 137. The World Bank. The pink column refers to the public expenditure as a % of the country's total healthcare expenditure. The blue dot is the country's expenditure on health per capita, expressed in international dollars at purchasing power parity.

The national infrastructure

India's National Health Policy (NHP) of 2017 set out to achieve the highest possible level of health and well-being for people of all ages, focusing on preventive and promotive healthcare, as well as universal access to quality health services without financial hardship.

To support this vision, the Ministry of Health and Family Welfare established a committee led by Shri J. Satyanarayana to develop an implementation framework for the National Health Stack. This effort resulted in the creation of the National Digital Health Blueprint (NDHB), which serves as the foundation for the country's digital health transformation.

Published in 2019, the NDHB outlines the context, rationale, scope, and implementation framework for building a nationwide digital healthcare ecosystem known as the Ayushman Bharat Digital Mission (ABDM). The NDHB's primary goals are to create an integrated digital health ecosystem, reduce out-of-pocket expenses, and achieve Universal Health Coverage (UHC).

The key objectives and proposals of the National Digital Health Blueprint (NDHB) are (Ministry of Health & Family Welfare, 2019):

Federated Architecture: information flows between different healthcare players, with decentralised data management at national, state, and facility levels. The aim is to ensure interoperability while maintaining flexibility in managing health data across the country.

Interoperability and Open Standards: adopting open standards and open-source software to facilitate interoperability between diverse health systems. Integration seeks both existing health information systems and new digital health initiatives smoothly, creating a unified ecosystem.

Patient-Centric Approach: citizens have full control over their health data, with privacy and data protection embedded into the system's design. Stringent security measures for data processing and storage are included to safeguard personal health information.

Core Building Blocks: The NDHB introduces key components such as Health IDs, Health Data Dictionaries, Electronic Health Records (EHR), and Personal Health Records (PHR). These core elements are designed to be minimalistic to ease adoption while building a unified health information infrastructure.

Integration of Health Services: The blueprint aims to integrate various national health programs, such as Ayushman Bharat, Reproductive Child Healthcare, and NIKSHAY (for tuberculosis), onto a unified IT platform. This integration is intended to enhance the efficiency of service delivery and ensure timely access to healthcare.

Stakeholder Collaboration: The NDHB encourages active participation and feedback from all stakeholders, including healthcare providers, technology developers, and the general public, to refine and effectively implement its digital health strategies.

Overview of the Federated Architecture of NDHB

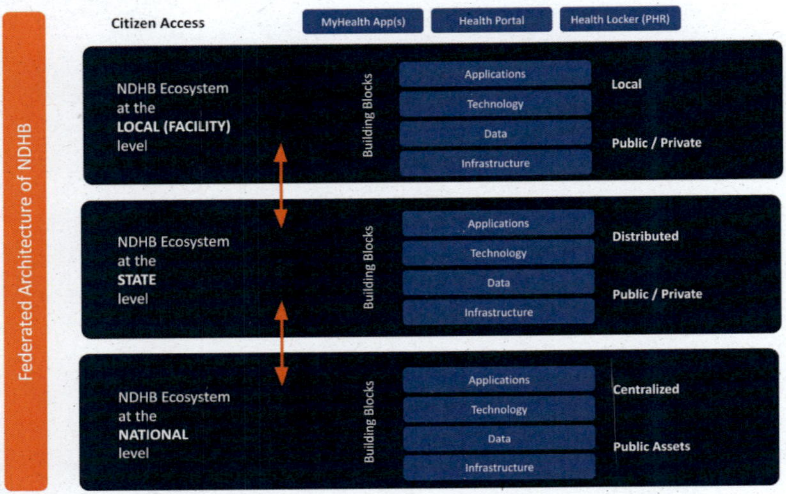

Figure 138. Ministry of Health. & Family Welfare, 2019. Page 14, Figure 2.1

The Ayushman Bharat Digital Mission (ABDM) presents a fascinating case as India's pioneering healthcare digital transformation project, mainly due to the country's vast population. According to *Forbes*, the scale and complexity of data management within ABDM could serve as a blueprint for other national health programs worldwide (Dans, 2020).

ABDM Technology Stack

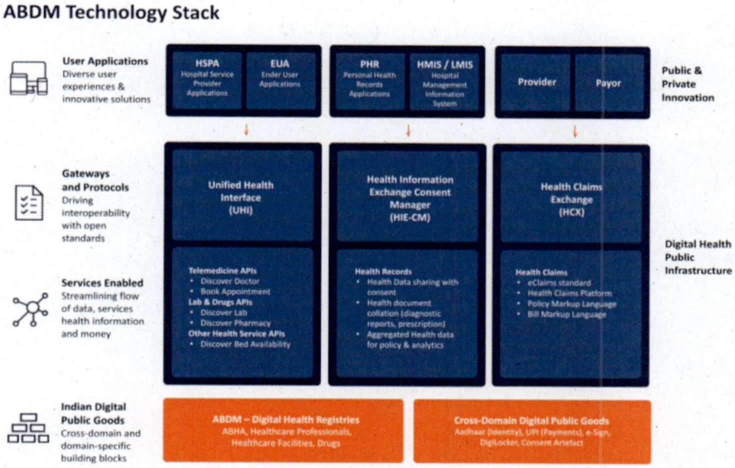

Figure 139. Presentation from the National Health Authority: "Introduction to Unified Health Interface (UHI)"

ABDM includes several health registries such as ABHA (a 14-digit patient identifier), HPR (Health Professional Registry), and HFR (Health Facility Registry). It will soon incorporate drug registries, enabling manufacturers to update and verify drugs through health authorities, allowing patients to check if a drug is unlicensed.

ABHA patient identifier

ABHA is a 14-digit unique identifier. Patients also create an ABHA address, similar to an email structure, which can be used to manage their healthcare data. While patients can create multiple ABHA addresses, they are uniquely identified within the healthcare ecosystem by their ABHA number. When a doctor shares healthcare records with a patient, they link it to the patient's preferred ABHA address, creating a part of their longitudinal health record.

ABHA leverages Aadhaar, a 12-digit unique identifier for Indian citizens, widely used in banking for KYC purposes. Although there are other methods for creating an ABHA (e.g., using a driving licence), Aadhaar allows for seamless, instant digital creation. Other methods require additional verification and authentication.

HPID professional identifier

Healthcare providers also have their own organisational IDs for each patient, and care providers are uniquely identified through the HPID (Health Professional ID).

ABDM interoperability gateways

The Ayushman Bharat Digital Mission (ABDM) relies on three key gateways and protocols to ensure interoperability through open standards: the Unified Health Interface (UHI), the Health Information Exchange Consent Manager (HIE-CM), and the Health Claims Exchange (HCX). Below is a more detailed explanation of each:

Unified Health Interface (UHI) clinical services

UHI facilitates various health services through Telemedicine APIs, including doctor discovery and appointment booking; Lab & Drugs APIs for discovering labs and pharmacies; and other Health Service APIs, such as checking bed availability in healthcare facilities.

User applications for Unified Health Interface(UHI) are Health Service Provider Applications (HSPA) and End User Application (EUA).

Health Information Exchange Consent Manager (HIE-CM) data movement, including for PHR

HIE-CM manages health records, enabling secure health data sharing with consent and facilitating the collation of health documents such as diagnostics, reports, and prescriptions. It also supports the aggregation of health data for policy and analytics purposes.

User applications for Health Information Exchange Consent Manager (HIE-CM) are Personal Health Records Applications (PHRs) and Hospital Management Information Systems (HMIS/LMIS).

Health Claims Exchange (HCX) policies and payments

HCX handles health claims using the cClaims standard and provides a platform for managing health claims, policy markup language, and bill markup language.

National PHRs

The National Health Authority (NHA) is the body responsible for steering ABDM. As part of this, it provides a certification framework for PHR applications. There are 3 stages of NHA compliance:

- **Milestone 1 (M1):** M1 signifies that a PHR application has met the initial compliance requirements necessary for certification. Specifically, this milestone focuses on enabling patients to verify their identity and create an ABHA.
- **Milestone 2 (M2):** at this stage, PHR applications must demonstrate the capability to manage patient health data securely. This includes storing, retrieving, and, in particular, sharing health records as needed. The application should be able to share data with other Health Information Providers (HIPs) and platforms using APIs.
- **Milestone 3 (M3):** to meet M3, the PHR has to develop Health Information User (HIU) services so that healthcare professionals can retrieve and view patients' data. In this system, when a doctor requests to pull a patient's data, a consent request is sent to the patient's app, allowing the doctor to access the necessary records. Patients can also

request to retrieve their own data from provider systems linked to their ABHA.

Below is a list of certified PHRs (the latest list is on this link: https://abdm.gov.in/our-partners/PHR):

- Plus ninety-one by Plus 91
- Driefcase, by Driefcase Health Tech Pvt Ltd
- Eka.care by Orbi Health Private Limited
- Paytm by Paytm
- Raxa by Raxa Health
- Arogya Setu by Arogya Setu
- Bajaj Finserv Health by Bajaj Finserv Health
- Parchaa by Panscience AI Healthcare Pvt Ltd
- Health-e by Anahat Solutions Pvt Ltd

Statistics

The following data has been retrieved on the 18th of November 2024 at 3 pm.

Ayushman Bharat Health Accounts (ABHA) created:

- 18th November 2024: 148,614
- November 2024: 5,672,874
- **Overall: 684,093,385**

Health Records Linked:

- 18th November 2024: 179,547
- November 2024: 6,596,401
- **Overall: 449,140,384**

ABHA accounts created, health records linked to ABHA accounts and new facilities using ABDM enabled software
January 2022 – November 2024

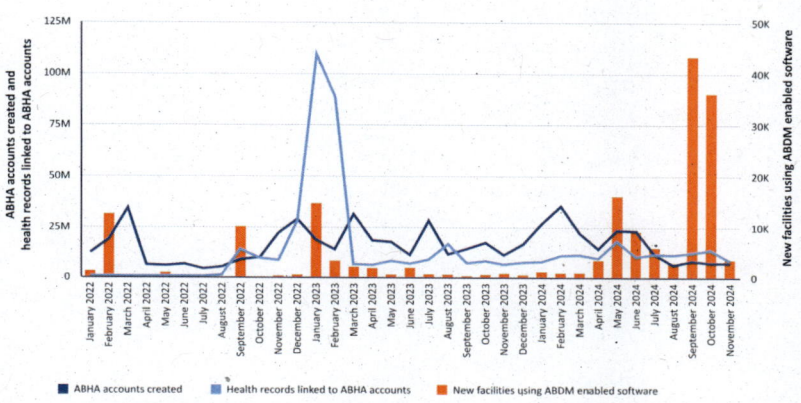

Figure 140. National Health Authority, Ministry of Health and Family Welfare, Government of India, 18th November 2024 - a; National Health Authority, Ministry of Health and Family Welfare, Government of India, 18th November 2024 - b.

Bibliography

- Ang, A., 2022. PHR app DRiefcase connects with India's ABDM. Healthcare IT News, 3 February. Available at: https://www.healthcareitnews.com/news/asia/phr-app-drief-case-connects-indias-abdm (accessed: 11 January 2024).

- Dans, E., 2020. How India's National Digital Health Mission Is Set To Revolutionize Healthcare. Forbes, updated 17 August. Available at: https://www.forbes.com/sites/en-riquedans/2020/08/17/how-indias-national-digital-health-mis-sion-is-set-to-revolutionize-healthcare/ (accessed: 11 January 2024).

- Driefcase Health-Tech, n.d. FAQs. Available at: https://drief-case.doctor/Faq.aspx (accessed: 11 January 2024).

- Driefcase Health-Tech, n.d. Homepage. Available at: https://www.driefcase.com/ (accessed: 11 January 2024).

- Matthan, R., 2023. The Third Way: India's Revolutionary Approach to Data Governance (accessed: 2 November 2024).

- Ministry of Health & Family Welfare, Government of India, 2019. National Digital Health Blueprint. Available at: https://abdm.gov.in:8081/uploads/ndhb_1_56ec695bc8.pdf (accessed: 20 July 2024).

- National Health Authority (NHA), Government of India, n.d. Ayushman Bharat Digital Mission (ABDM). Available at: https://abdm.gov.in/ (accessed: 11 January 2024).

- NITI Aayog, 2021. Health Insurance for India's Missing Middle. Available at: https://www.niti.gov.in/sites/default/files/2021-10/HealthInsurance-forIndiasMissingMiddle_28-10-2021.pdf (accessed: 20 August 2024).

- Tikkanen, R., Osborn, R., Mossialos, E., Djordjevic, A., & Wharton, G.A., 2020. International Health Care System Profiles: India. The Commonwealth Fund. Available at: https://www.commonwealthfund.org/international-health-policy-center/countries/india (accessed: 26 July 2024).

INDIA – DRIEFCASE

The PHR

DRiefcase is India's first and largest licensed Personal Health Record (PHR). The National Health Authority (NHA) approved it in 2022 for the roll-out of the Ayushman Bharat Digital Mission (ABDM).

PHR: The DRiefcase Health Locker app allows users and their families to securely store and access medical records anytime and from anywhere. With a focus on personal health records management, the app offers easy upload and quick retrieval of patient data, enabling safe remote care. To access and share health records digitally, users need an ABHA account (formerly known as Health ID), which serves as a unique health identifier. Premium versions of the app offer additional features.

EHR: DRiefcase also offers a clinic management system for doctors and healthcare providers called DRiefcase Connect. This is a practice management platform for individual doctors, polyclinics, and small hospitals, designed to enhance productivity for healthcare professionals (DRiefcase Health-Tech, 2024-a).

History

DRiefcase was founded in 2016 by Sohit Kapoor and Harsh Parikh, both former investment bankers motivated by their personal experiences with the healthcare system. Observing the inefficiencies and paperwork in healthcare, they wanted to bring the advancements seen in financial services. As healthcare data is scattered across multiple providers in India, they believed patients should be the central decision-makers and aggregators of their own healthcare information. This vision led to the creation of DRiefcase as a PHR. Quick and easy access to medical histories would simplify the burden of health records management and bridge the information gap between patients and doctors.

Digital health was still in its infancy in India, with national conversations only beginning in 2017. Despite early challenges, the founders funded DRiefcase and gradually expanded its capabilities and user base.

The company's first working release was a basic storage platform for photographs of medical records. Next was a rapid data retrieval feature, essential for India's short consultations with doctors.

India has evolved, with many records now digital and citizens able to create a unique digital identifier for health (ABHA). DRiefcase links patient records to their ABHA accounts. A governmental directive requests all providers to connect to the ABDM framework by 2027.

In February 2022, India's National Health Authority approved the integration of DRiefcase with the ABDM, enabling DRiefcase to launch a faster check-in service (PKB interviews, 2024).

Features

The primary use of the platform involves functionalities related to the ABDM, such as the creation of an ABHA, management of consent and health records, and the ability for individuals to scan or capture images of their health documents for uploading. Patients can share their records with doctors (DRiefcase Health-Tech, 2024-a; PKB interviews, 2024).

PHR

Patients can input their own information and access data entered by doctors into an ABDM-compliant EHR (such as DRiefcase'a Connect).

Patients can upload radiology, pathology, and laboratory reports. They can also take notes about their health in a journal.

DRiefcase automatically tags and indexes to quickly locate and retrieve any record.

Patients can create profiles for family members within a single account. (DRiefcase Health-Tech, 2024-a; PKB interviews, 2024).

EHR

Doctors using DRiefcase Connect (the EHR product) can share records with patients (DRiefcase Health-Tech, 2024-a; PKB interviews, 2024). Each patient will have access to:

- Diagnoses, medication, and immunisations
- Procedure history
- Appointments (with reminders) and the ability to book new appointments
- Video consultations

Ask for blood donors

"Call for Blood" is designed to address the critical need for timely blood donations during medical emergencies. Launched in December 2023, "users seeking blood within a city can connect with willing donors through the app. This is not just an app feature; it's a lifeline for those in need. Our goal is to save lives and ensure that vital resources are always at hand." (Harsh Parikh, Co-Founder of DRiefcase, PKB interviews.)

The 'Call for Blood' icon asks the user to provide essential details, including name, blood group, contact information, and location. DRiefcase will notify other users in the same geographical area (Business Standard, 2023).

Screenshots

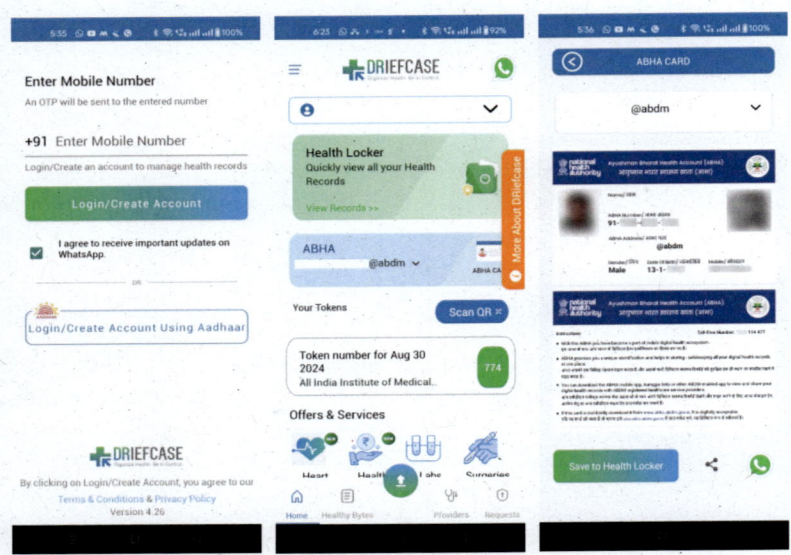

Figure 141. Login page. Patients have the option to log in or create an account using Aadhaar (the national 12-digit biometric identifier).

Figure 142. Homepage once logged in.

Figure 143. Patients can use their ABHA Card on DRiefcase for checking in quickly at a health care facility.

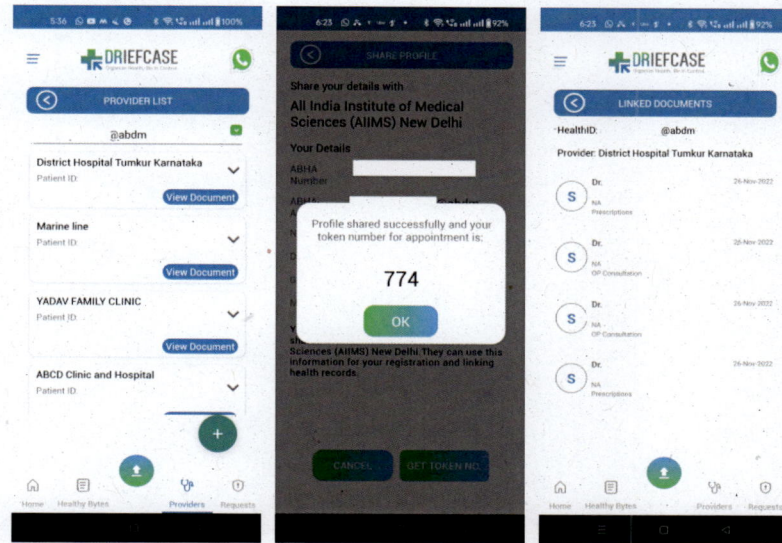

Figure 144. Patients can see a list of providers and health documents about them from each provider.

Figure 145. Patients can scan a QR code and register with the hospital seamlessly. This process would otherwise take 4 - 6 hours.

Figure 146. Patients can view records linked by any provider.

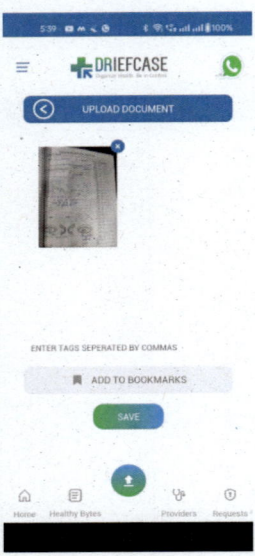

Figure 147. Patients can upload their health documents to their records, for example, scanning them or taking pictures.

Revenues

Scanning

"Scan at Home" helps people digitise their paper medical notes. Scanning is free if the user sends and picks up the paper. Alternatively, a team can visit homes to scan for ₹1,000, about $12 (DRiefcase Health-Tech, 2024-b):

- DRiefcase can collect medical documents from the patient's premises, scan them centrally, and return them to the patient. This costs ₹1,000 and is available throughout India.

- DRiefcase can scan and upload medical documents at the patient's premises. This costs ₹1,000 and is available in select Indian cities.
- DRiefcase can send a flash drive or CD with a copy of the data it scanned. This costs ₹1,000 and is available across India.

Commissions for transactions

DRiefcase earns commissions on services booked through the platform. Launched in June 2024, the company and its partners provide services such as pathology, health loans, insurance, and teleconsultations (PKB interviews, 2024).

Published outcomes - statistics

As of August 2024, DRiefcase has 16 million registered users (PKB interviews, 2024). Each day, 80,000 patients register for an ABHA ID through DRiefcase, aided by informative posters in hospitals and on-site interns stationed in 150 hospitals across India. The user acquisition cost remains notably low at a few cents per user.

To better understand these figures, it's helpful to consider them in the context of India's broader statistics:

Currently, around 600 million Indians possess ABHA IDs. Government programmes generated 80% of these without patients being aware of their existence. Only 80 to 100 million of the total AHBD IDs were voluntarily created by citizens. Each day, 250,000 people either register for or use their ABHA IDs.

DRiefcase's users are 50% of these 250,000 daily users, either for registering or returning visits (PKB interviews, 2024).

Challenges and areas for improvement

Despite its many successes, DRiefcase faces several challenges. A significant one is the adoption and data flow of the ABHA ID system by healthcare providers, which relies heavily on the federal government's management.

DRiefcase only receives between 25,000 and 30,000 patient records daily from the 80,000 new users registering each day. Furthermore, these records primarily consist of PDFs and basic consultation summaries. For many patients, data from hospitals is still not flowing seamlessly.

Monetisation is difficult, even while the app has captured 50% of India's market. The company has not yet fully calculated the Return on Investment (ROI) or the lifetime value of its users, as it only recently launched its healthcare services, such as pathology and health loans (PKB interviews, 2024).

Bibliography

- Business Standard, 2023. DRiefcase Launches a New App Feature - Call for Blood: Connecting Donors and Patients in Need. 2 December. Available at: https://www.business-standard.com/content/press-releases-ani/driefcase-launches-a-new-app-feature-call-for-blood-connecting-donors-and-patients-in-need-123120200591_1.html (accessed: 26 July 2024).

- DRiefcase Health-Tech, 2024-a, Homepage. Available at: https://www.driefcase.com/ (accessed: 11 January 2024).

- DRiefcase Health-Tech, 2024-c, FAQs. Available at: https://driefcase.doctor/Faq.aspx (accessed: 11 January 2024).

- DRiefcase Health-Tech, 2024-b, Premium Services. Available at: https://www.driefcase.com/premium-scanning-services/ (accessed: 11 January 2024).

ITALY

Dr Maria Montessori was appointed co-director of Rome's new Scuola Ortofrénica, dedicated to training teachers to work with children who had cognitive and developmental challenges. Starting in 1899, her techniques helped children with difficulties catch up with those without. So she wondered how much regular schooling was holding back normal children. Montessori schools eventually taught many technology founders, including Larry Page and Sergey Brin (Google), Jeff Bezos (Amazon), and Jimmy Wales (Wikipedia).

Country's healthcare system in a nutshell

Italy's regionalised National Health Service (Servizio Sanitario Nazionale, SSN) has provided universal coverage to all citizens and legal residents since 1978. The SSN is organised under the national Ministry of Health and administered on a regional basis. The central government establishes the national benefits package and allocates funding to the regions. The regions are responsible for financing, planning, and delivering healthcare services at the local level.

The SSN is primarily funded through a combination of regional and national taxes, with pooled funds managed at the national level. Each region's share of funding is determined by a formula that takes into account epidemiological factors such as population age structure. This formula is agreed annually between the national government and the regions at the State-Regions Conference, an intergovernmental forum for decision-making. The national government provides additional financial support through an equalisation fund, sourced from national value-added tax, to cover the gap between each region's estimated financial needs and its own revenue.

Out-of-pocket (OOP) payments in Italy are significantly higher than the EU's average. In 2019, Italy's OOP accounted for 23.3% of total health expenditure, while the EU average was 15.4%. The majority of OOP spending in Italy goes towards direct payments for services not covered by the SSN, particularly outpatient medical care and over-the-counter medications. The remaining OOPs are co-payments for covered services such as medications, outpatient specialist visits, and diagnostic tests (World Health Organization, 2022).

Health insurance covers the entire population of Italy. This encompasses both those who are members of health insurance schemes and those who have free access to state-provided healthcare services (Our World in Data, n.p.).

Public vs private

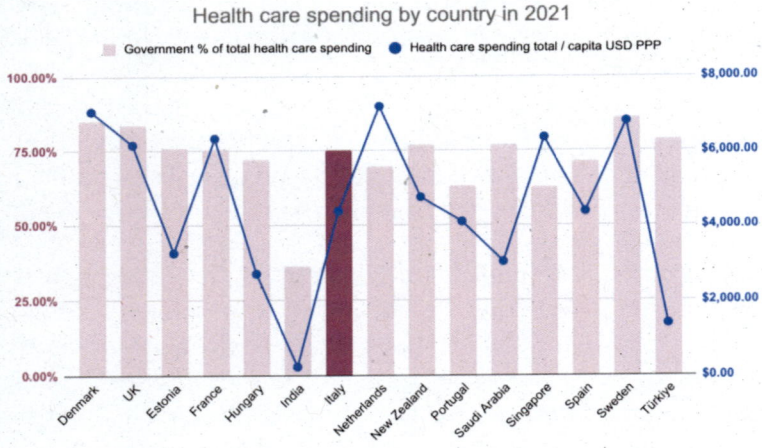

Figure 148. Source: The World Bank. The pink column refers to the public expenditure as a % of the country's total healthcare expenditure. The blue dot is the country's expenditure on health per capita, expressed in international dollars at purchasing power parity.

The national PHR

History

Fascicolo Sanitario Elettronico (FSE), the Italian National PHR, was introduced from Art. 12 of Law Decree 18 Oct 2012 n. 179. The law established that:

Each region had to create and implement a PHR by June 20, 2015.

The user interfaces, systems, and software must ensure full interoperability at regional, national, and European levels.

Some regions had started local FSE projects before this law, such as the Emilia Romagna region (Posteraro, 2021).

In more recent years, Italy wrote, as requested by the EU recovery package Next Generation EU (NGEU), the National Plan of Recovery and Resilience (PNRR), in which each country has to define a plan of reforms and investments for the period 2021-2026. The Italian PNRR was officially approved by the Italian Government on the 13th of July 2021.

Italy's National Plan of Recovery and Resilience (PNRR) allocated 2.5 billion euros for digital health, with 1.3 billion euros dedicated to establishing a national data infrastructure for the FSE. The infrastructure aims to be homogeneous across the country and to include the entire clinical history of patients. The budget is for 2021-2026 (Permanent Conference for Relations between the State, the Regions, and the Autonomous Provinces, 2022).

Region	Who built the PHR	Public / Private
Abruzzo	Has not developed its FSE. According to the 'subsidiarity regime,' the region is using the nationally available infrastructure with basic features.	-
Basilicata	Region Basilicata	Built In-house.
Bolzano (autonomous province)	Autonmous province of Bolzano	Built In-house.
Calabria	Has not developed its FSE. According to the 'subsidiarity regime,' the region is using the nationally available infrastructure with basic features.	-
Campania	Has not developed its FSE. According to the 'subsidiarity regime,' the region is using the nationally available infrastructure with basic features.	-
Emilia-Romagna	Lepida	Region is main shareholder.
Friuli Venezia Giulia	Insiel	Company owned by the region.
Lazio	Engineering Ingegneria Informatica - won tender in 2015	Private company.

Liguria	Liguria Digitale	Region is main shareholder.
Lombardia	Lombardia Informatica	The region is the main shareholder.
Marche	Cineca	Cineca is a non-profit consortium made up of 69 Italian universities, 27 national public research centres, the Italian Ministry of Universities and Research, and the Italian Ministry of Education.
Molise	Under development, no specified company.	
Piemonte	CSI Piemonte	Consortium of public entities.
Puglia	Innovapuglia	Region is main shareholder.
Sardegna	Almaviva	Private company.
Sicilia	Has not developed its FSE. According to the 'subsidiarity regime,' the region is using the nationally available infrastructure with basic features.	
Toscana	Dedalus	Private company.
Trento (autonomous province)	Trentino Network	Region is main shareholder.

Umbria	Region Umbria	Built In-house.
Valle D'Aosta	Region Valle d'Aosta	Built In-house.
Veneto	Consorzio Arsenàl.IT	Public consortium of the 9 Local Health Authorities and the 2 Hospital Companies of the Region. The regional government, through its health structures, is the main shareholder of the consortium.

Features

Regional Fascicolo Sanitario Elettronico (FSE) systems must adhere to the national minimum standards for data sharing and basic features. However, each FSE is still distinct, with variation across regions, and it is, therefore, difficult to define a uniform set of features.

The core elements of the FSE, as stated in the national legislation, include patient demographics, clinical reports (e.g., specialist visit reports, test results, radiology), A&E reports, discharge letters, organ donation consent, a patient summary, and pharmaceutical dossier.

The pharmaceutical dossier is updated by pharmacies. It helps track a patient's medication history, assess the appropriateness of new prescriptions, and monitor adherence to therapies. However, this feature is still underdeveloped in many regions.

The patient summary provides a concise overview of the patient's clinical profile, including chronic conditions, transplants, adverse drug reactions, and allergies. It is created by the GP or paediatrician and is particularly useful in emergencies, offering clinicians a quick snapshot of the patient's health. Despite its importance, GPs have been slow to adopt this feature, citing the time-consuming nature of creating the summary, the lack of direct benefit to their own practice, and concerns about being held accountable for medical decisions made by other clinicians based on this information.

In addition to these core features, regions may choose to include optional elements in their FSE. These can include:

- Patient ability to add notes and clinical documents, which promotes self-management and empowerment. Some argue that this should become a core feature.
- In-home assistance programs.
- Care plans.
- Medical certificates.
- Vaccination records.

Recent legislation, the Decreto Rilancio (2020), mandates the integration of the FSE with other national systems (Posteraro, 2021), including:

- The Transplants Information System (Sistema Informativo Trapianti - SIT), a digital platform for managing data related to the National Transplants Network.
- The Italian Vaccine Registry.
- Regional appointment management systems (CUPs).

Challenges and areas for improvement

Over the past decade, several regions in Italy have initiated projects to develop platforms for collecting clinical records produced by their healthcare institutions. However, differences in processes, architectural models, and technological advancements across these regions have prevented the achievement of true interoperability (Ciampi et al., 2019).

Each region establishes its own Fascicolo Sanitario Elettronico (FSE), following a model based on a network of regional systems rather than a unified national system. Therefore, currently, patients can only access their FSE through the platform provided by their region. This creates challenges when they move to a different region, as they may need to adopt a new access method, potentially finding it difficult or impossible to retrieve their previous records.

A law from 2015 mandated that each region implement the FSE using a technological infrastructure interoperable with other regional FSEs, ensuring that patients could move between regions without losing access to their data. To achieve this, in 2018, the National Infrastructure for Interoperability (INI) was introduced, aiming to transition from a federated system to a centralized national one with a single point of access. However, this centralization has not yet been realized.

Currently, interoperability remains ineffective due to several factors (Posteraro, 2021):

- Data heterogeneity across regions
- The use of different technological standards
- The existence of varying regional laws

In 2023, Carlo De Masi, president of the Italian National Consumers Protection Association, remarked that the lack of interoperability between regional systems not only compromises patient safety but also diminishes the FSE's overall utility and effectiveness (CISL, 2023).

New architecture:

In 2022, guidelines for the creation of a more integrated FSE were published in the Gazzetta Ufficiale della Repubblica Italiana (the official journal of record for the Italian government). The diagram below illustrates the existing regional registries and an interoperability platform (shown in dark purple) alongside the proposed future interventions (in purple). Despite having regional registries and a platform for interoperability, the absence of a central data repository, a national registry, and structured data (ideally in FHIR format) renders the current interoperability platform largely unusable.

FSE Architecture

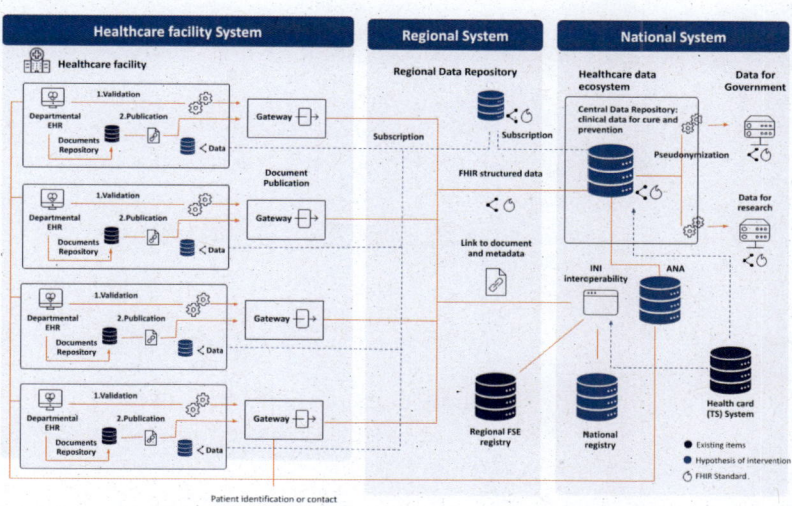

Figure 149. 'Guidelines for the creation of the FSE' (Gazzetta Ufficiale della repubblica Italiana 11-07-2022).

Published outcomes - statistics

As of the third trimester of 2023, nearly all Italian citizens have activated their Fascicolo Sanitario Elettronico (FSE), with 57.66 million users out of a total population of 58.85 million. However, login and usage rates remain low.

Patient Utilisation:

- Only in one region (Emilia Romagna) did more than 50% of citizens use the FSE.
- In seven regions, less than 20% of patients accessed their FSE.
- In nine regions, 0% of patients utilized the FSE.

Clinician Utilisation:

- In five regions, 0% of clinicians used the FSE.
- In seven regions, less than 50% of clinicians accessed the platform.
- Only in two regions did clinicians add information to the "patient summary."

Healthcare Facility Participation:

- In 10 regions (including one autonomous province), no healthcare facilities contributed data to their citizens' FSE.
- In six regions, less than 60% of healthcare facilities participated.
- Only in four regions did more than 60% of facilities add data to the FSE.

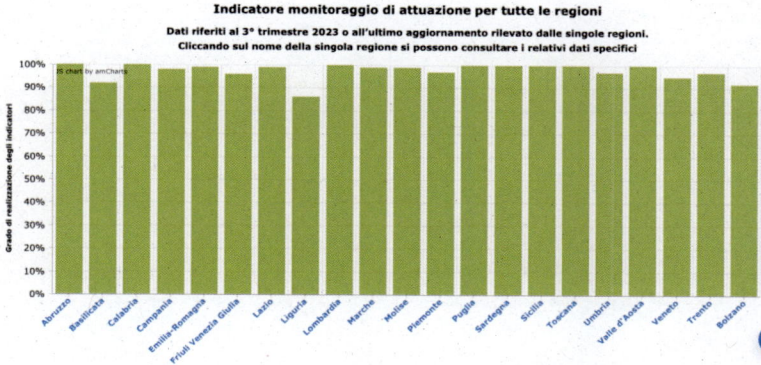

Figure 150. Implementation indicators in the various regions. It checks the pro-gress of regional realisation of the Electronic Health Record. 3rd trimester of 2023.

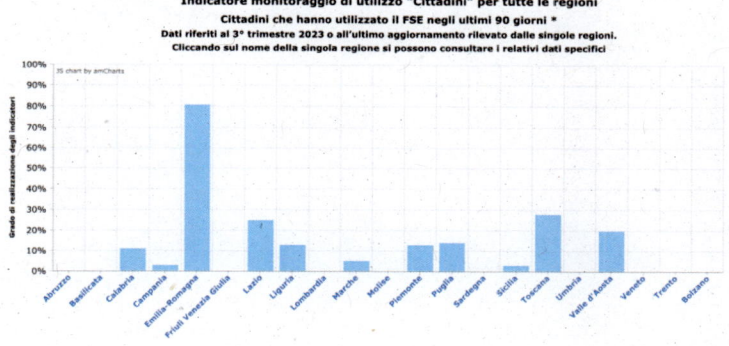

Figure 151. Percentage of access in each region by patients that had at least 1 new data added to their record in the last 90 days. 3rd trimester of 2023.

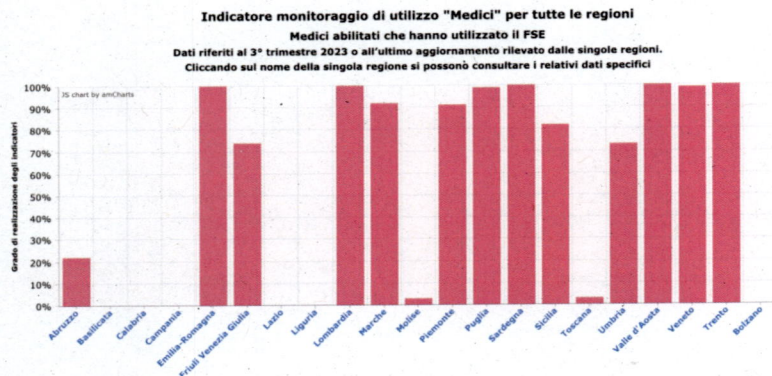

Figure 152. Percentage of clinicians who accessed the FSE. 3rd trimester of 2023.

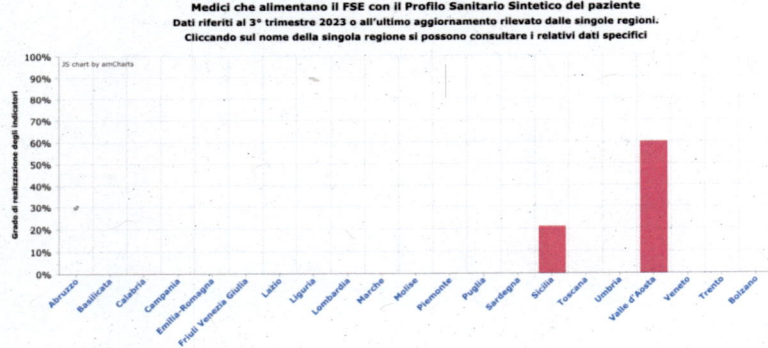

Figure 153. Percentage of clinicians who added data to the 'Patient Summary' per region. 3rd trimester of 2023.

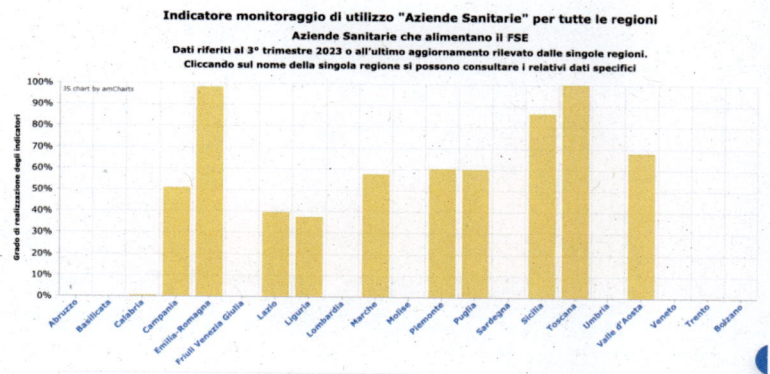

Figure 154. Percentage of healthcare facilities that add data to the FSE for their patients per region. 3rd trimester of 2023.

([AGID Agenzia per l'Italia Digitale, 2023-2024](#))

As of May 2024, the Government has released new statistics on the percentage of Regions and Autonomous Provinces where the FSE is configured to store specific types of documents. However, while the system is capable of storing these documents, their actual presence in a patient's record depends on the particular healthcare facility involved. All of them are configured to store discharge letters, prescriptions, referrals, lab results, imaging results, outpatient appointment reports, and emergency admission reports. More than half also have pathology reports, patient summaries, vaccination certificates, documents attesting specialist care service have been provided, documents attesting the prescribed medication has been bought, and personal health diaries.

Statistics regarding other services offered through the FSEs are also available. In 95% of the regions, the FSEs are configured to display the COVID-19 certificate. More than half of the regions allow patients to request exemption certificates for service fees through their PHRs (81%), make co-payments for services (76%), book appointments with specialists in public healthcare facilities upon referral (76%), choose and change general practitioners (76%). In

48% of the Regions, patients can also invite carers to view their records.

(AGID Agenzia per l'Italia Digitale, 2023-2024)

Screenshots

The below screenshots refer to the PHR in the Emilia-Romagna region in Italy created by Lepida. As of August 2024, the region has the highest PHR usage in Italy.

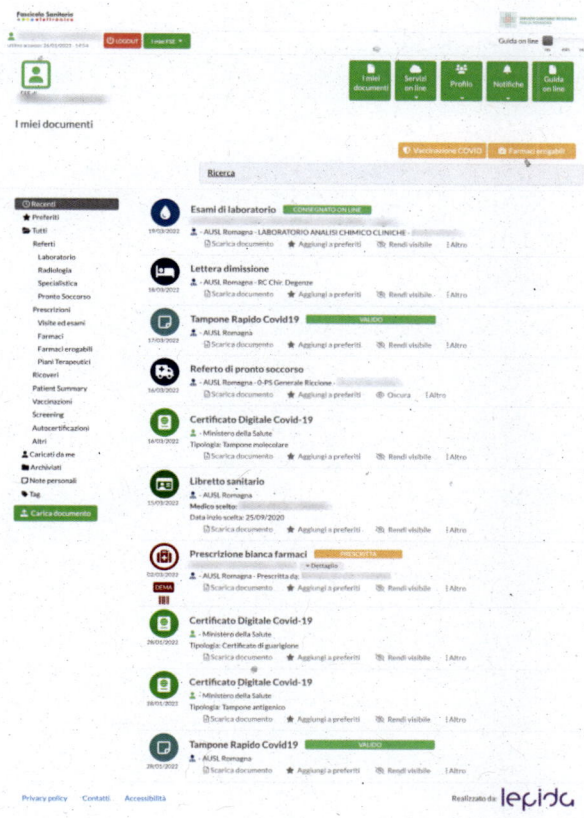

Figure 155. The home page of the Emilia Romagna region FSE provides an overview of the patient's interactions with the national health service, organised by the most recent activities. This includes, among others, lab results, admission and discharge letters, and medical prescriptions. On the left side, patients can access a menu that includes various sections. The Recent tab displays the latest interactions, while the Preferred tab allows patients to quickly access health documents that they have starred. The All option presents a complete list of interactions. Patients can find detailed Reports encompassing tests, radiology, specialty medicine, and A&E visits. The Prescriptions section includes information on appointments and exams, medications, deliverable medicines, care plans, and admissions. Additional features such as the Patient Summary, vaccinations, screening, self-certifications, and others are also available. Patients can contribute to their records with the Contributed by Me option, manage archived information, and take personal notes. Finally, the menu allows patients to tag specific entries and upload documents.

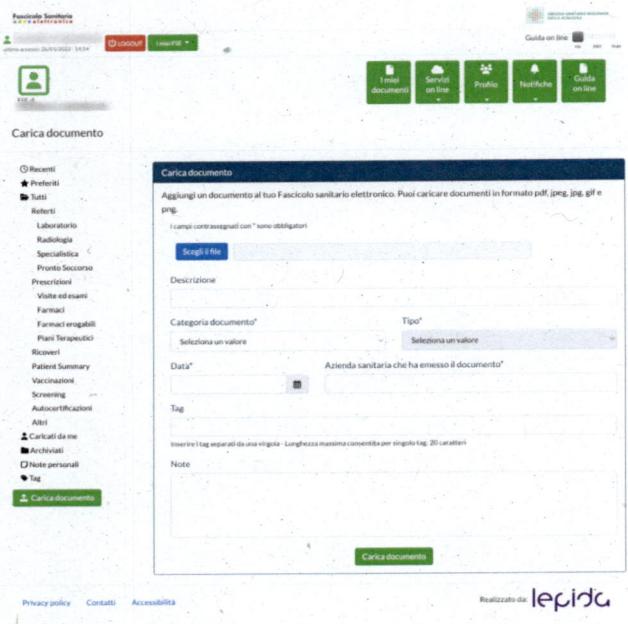

Figure 156. The Upload Document feature allows patients to add various file types, including PDF, JPEG, JPG, GIF, and PNG. Patients can provide a description for each document. Additionally, they can select the type of document, such as discharge or admission letters, and specify the healthcare provider that initially created the document.

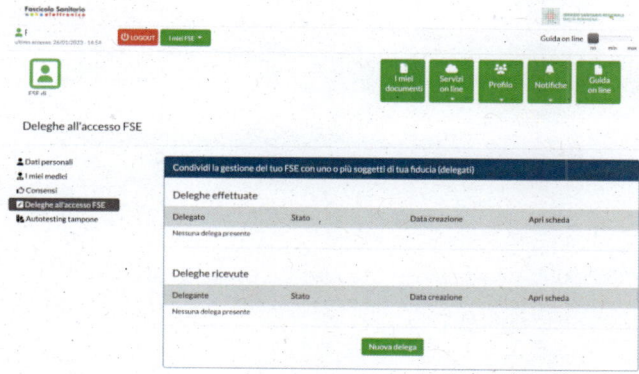

Figure 157. The Delegates page is designed for patients to add trustees or carers to their health records. The menu on the left, titled "Delegations for FSE Access," provides access to various sections. Patients can view their Personal Data, which outlines the information associated with their account. The My Clinicians section lists the healthcare professionals involved in their care, while the Consents page details any permissions granted. In the Delegations section, patients can share the management of their record with one or more individuals of their choosing, re-ferred to as delegates. Additionally, the Auto Testing section provides information related to COVID testing.

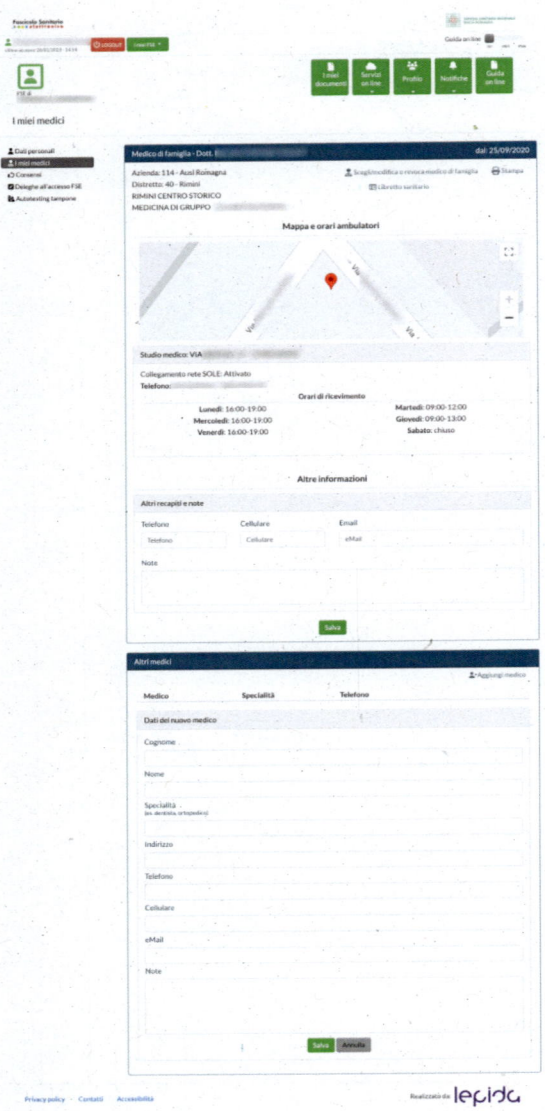

Figure 158. The My Clinicians page provides patients with information about their healthcare professionals, including their GP. This section displays the GP's address, office hours, telephone number, and a map. Patients have the option to change their GP directly from this page. Additionally, at the bottom of the page, patients can add other professionals of their choice.

160

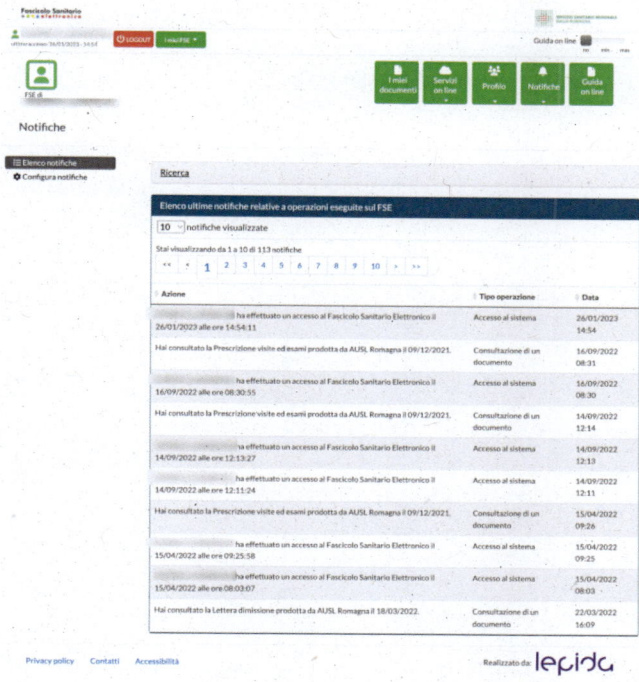

Figure 159. The Notifications Page provides patients with a list of those who have accessed their health records. It indicates whether the individual consulted a document and specifies which document was viewed. Each entry is timestamped, displaying the date and time of access.

Bibliography

- AGID Agenzia Per l'Italia Digitale, n.d. Fascicolo Sanitario Elettronico - Monitoring. Available at: https://www.fascicolosanitario.gov.it/en/monitoring (accessed: 29 April 2024).

- Ciampi, M., Esposito, A. and Sicuranza, M., n.d. Stato dell'arte sulle iniziative nazionali relative allo sviluppo di sistemi ICT interoperabili per la Salute Digitale. Available at: https://www.researchgate.net/profile/Mario-Ciampi/publication/334204495_Stato_dell'arte_sulle_iniziative_nazionali_relative_allo_sviluppo_di_sistemi_ICT_interoperabili_per_la_Sa-lute_Digitale/links/5d1cc763299bf1547c94fbd3/Stato-dellarte-sulle-iniziative-nazionali-relative-allo-sviluppo-di-sistemi-ICT-in-teroperabili-per-la-Salute-Digitale.pdf (accessed: 29 April 2024).

- CISL, 2023. Consumatori. Adiconsum Cisl: "The Current Electronic Health Record Without Interoperability Does Not Protect Citizens' Health and Increases Healthcare Costs, Making the Tool Useless and Ineffective". (online) 26 January. Available at: https://www.cisl.it/notizie/categorie-ed-enti-cisl/consumatori-adiconsum-cisl-lattuale-fascicolo-sanitario-elettronico-senza-in-teroperabilita-non-tutela-la-salute-dei-cittadini-consumatori-e-fa-lievitare-i-costi-della-sanita-rende/ (accessed: 29 April 2024).

- Gazzetta Ufficiale della Repubblica Italiana, 2022, 11 July. FSE (Allegato A). Gazzetta Ufficiale della Repubblica Italiana, Serie generale - n. 160, 11-07-2022. Available at: https://www.gazzettauffi-ciale.it/eli/id/2022/07/11/22A03961/sg (accessed: 29 April 2024).

- Permanent Conference for Relations between the State, the Regions, and the Autonomous Provinces, 2022. Digital Health. Presentation to the Permanent Conference for Relations between the State, the Regions, and the Autonomous Provinces, Rome, 2 March 2022. REP. ATTI No. 22/CSR of 2 March 2022. Available at: https://www.statoregioni.it/it/conferenza-stato-regioni/sedute-2022/seduta-del-02032022/atti/repertorio-atto-n-22csr/ (accessed: 29 April 2024).

- Posteraro, N., 2021. La digitalizzazione della sanità in Italia: uno sguardo al Fascicolo Sanitario Elettronico (anche alla luce del PNRR). FEDERALISMI. IT, 2021, pp.1-42. Available at: https://air.unimi.it/handle/2434/946488 (accessed: 29 April 2024).

- World Health Organization, 2022. Italy: health system review. Health Systems in Transition, 24(4). Available at: https://euro-healthobservatory.who.int/publications/i/italy-health-system-review-2022 (accessed: 29 April 2024).

NETHERLANDS

The Dutch pioneered using private markets to solve public prob-
lems. Amsterdam's stock exchange in 1602 was the first in the
world; its first listing was the Dutch East India Company, the first
multinational company in the world; the Dutch dairy industry is
highly competitive, leading to global exports; the country was an
early deregulator of telecoms, exposing its national telecoms
champion to competition; the Royal FloraHolland auction system is
one of the most competitive and efficient in the world so the country handles 60% of the world's flower exports.

Therefore, its approach to personal health records is the opposite
of that of neighbouring Denmark and statist France. It avoided a
single offering and instead opened up a competitive market.

Country's healthcare system in a nutshell

In the Netherlands, the healthcare system combines public funding
with private insurance. Every resident must obtain statutory health
insurance from private insurers, who are mandated to accept all
applicants. The system is mainly funded through public sources, including premiums, taxes, and government grants. The national government sets healthcare priorities and oversees aspects of access,
quality, and costs. Standard benefits include hospital care, physician services, home nursing, mental health care, and prescription
medications. While adults are responsible for paying premiums,
annual deductibles, and coinsurance or copayments for certain services and drugs, the government covers healthcare costs for children up to the age of 18.

Municipalities manage specific health services, such as preventive
screenings and outpatient long-term care. The Federal Ministry of

Health takes on a regulatory role rather than managing healthcare directly.

Several independent bodies set operational priorities:

- The Health Council provides guidance to the government on evidence-based medicine, public health, and environmental protection.
- The Medicines Evaluation Board ensures the efficacy, safety, and quality of medicines.
- The National Health Care Institute evaluates new technologies for effectiveness and cost and advises on their inclusion in the mandatory benefit package.
- The Dutch Health Care Authority oversees the functioning of health insurance, purchasing, and care delivery markets.
- The Dutch Competition Authority enforces competition laws among insurers and providers.
- The Health Care Inspectorate monitors the quality, safety, and accessibility of care. Self-regulation by medical professionals is also a key element of the system.

Health information technology (IT) is not centralised. The Union of Providers for Health Care Communication manages the data exchange through IT infrastructure (Tikkanen et al., 2020).

According to the most recent data from 2010, health insurance covered 98.9% of the population in the Netherlands. This coverage encompasses both those who are members of health insurance schemes and those who have free access to state-provided healthcare services (Our World in Data, n.p.).

Public vs private

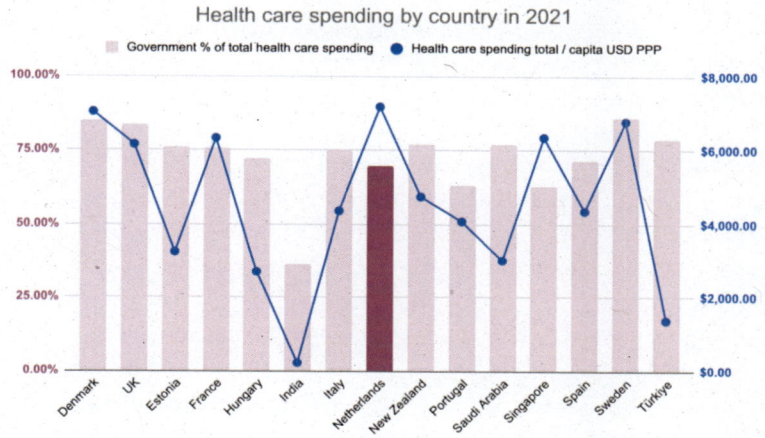

Figure 160. Source: The World Bank. The pink column refers to the public expenditure as a % of the country's total healthcare expenditure. The blue dot is the country's expenditure on health per capita, expressed in international dollars at purchasing power parity.

The national PHR

History

In 2011, initial discussions began in the Netherlands about creating a national Electronic Patient File (EPD), which would standardise medical records for every patient and enable them to access their medical data. However, this project failed to gain support from the Senate.

In response, the Dutch Patient Federation introduced an alternative solution: MedMij and the personal health environment (PGO) (PGO.nl, 2023). The MedMij foundation was established in 2015 by the Informatieberaad Zorg (Healthcare Information Council), a collaborative body involving various stakeholders from the healthcare sector and the Ministry of Health, Welfare, and Sport. This initiative, led by the Patiëntenfederatie Nederland (Dutch Patients Federation), aims to set standards for the secure exchange of health data in the Netherlands.

Currently, MedMij represents the benchmark for the secure transmission of health data between patients and healthcare providers. Organisations that meet the stringent criteria set by MedMij are authorised to use its label. This certification ensures that individuals can access their health data through a PGO of their choosing. The MedMij label denotes adherence to the standards outlined in the MedMij Framework. It is awarded to apps, websites, or PGOs that meet these requirements and is also displayed at healthcare providers' locations that participate in the MedMij network.

While the MedMij label guarantees secure data exchange, it does not provide information about the functionality or user-friendliness of the certified tools. Patients are responsible for selecting the app or website that best suits their needs (MedMij, 2023).

As of January 2025, there are 16 PGOs that meet MedMij standards, offering patients a choice of platforms. An updated list is available on the MedMij Participants web page.

Investments

The Dutch Ministry of Health, Welfare, and Sport (VWS) has made significant investments in healthcare digitalisation in recent years. One of the major initiatives is the Dutch Health Information Council, which oversees the National Health Information Exchange Infrastructure (VIPP) program. This program has received substantial funding to improve digital information exchange across healthcare providers, enhancing patient care and efficiency (VIPPGGZ, n.d.).

In total, the VWS has allocated around €900 million to various digital health initiatives. The VIPP program itself was initially funded with €400 million, aimed at upgrading hospital information systems, improving patient access to medical records, and facilitating inter-organisational data exchange. Of this, hospitals (VIPP 1) received €105 million, while GPs were allocated €75 million (PKB interviews, 2024).

Additionally, €75 million has been earmarked for artificial intelligence in healthcare and digital innovation, focusing on areas such as telehealth, digital diagnostics, and personalised medicine. These investments are part of a broader strategy to modernise the healthcare system, making it more resilient and efficient through technology.

Overall, the VWS's efforts reflect a strong commitment to integrating digital solutions within the healthcare sector, aiming to improve efficiency and support population health management.

Bibliography

- MedMij, 2023. About MedMij (online) Available at: https://medmij.nl/en/home/ (accessed: 2 November 2023).

- MedMij, 2023. MedMij participants (online) Available at: https://medmij.nl/medmij-deelnemers/ (accessed: 2 November 2023).

- PGO, 2023. What is a PGO? (online) Available at: https://www.pgo.nl/wat-is-een-pgo/ (accessed: 2 November 2023).

- Tikkanen, R., Osborn, R., Mossialos, E., Djordjevic, A. and Wharton, G.A., 2020. International Health Policy Center: Netherlands. The Commonwealth Fund. Available at: https://www.commonwealthfund.org/international-health-policy-center/countries/netherlands (accessed: 2 November 2023).

- VIPPGGZ, n.d. Regulation. The State Secretary of Health, Welfare and Sport. Available at: https://www-vippggz-nl.translate.goog/regeling.html?_x_tr_sl=nl&_x_tr_tl=en&_x_tr_hl=en&_x_tr_pto=sc (accessed: 3 September 2024).

NEW ZEALAND

New Zealand is far away but far ahead. It was the first to have universal women's suffrage (1893), national minimum wage (1894), and universal pension (1898). Prime Minister Jacinda Ardern delivered the world's first wellbeing budget in 2019, some of the lowest excess death rates during Covid, and her legislation to prevent a new generation from buying cigarettes was copied by the British government when she stepped down in New Zealand.

Country's healthcare system in a nutshell

New Zealand's healthcare system, overseen by Te Whatu Ora - Health New Zealand, is of high quality and largely funded through general taxation. This funding model ensures that healthcare services are either free or subsidised for those eligible for publicly funded healthcare. For instance, public hospitals provide free treatment to citizens and permanent residents, while primary care services and medications listed by PHARMAC (the government agency managing the pharmaceutical budget) are subsidised. Patients are still required to make a co-payment.

Although the public system covers most healthcare needs, private health insurance is available to expedite access to specific treatments (Southern Health, n.d.). Emergency services are primarily provided by St John New Zealand, a charity operated by volunteers and funded through a mix of private donations and public subsidies (Givealittle, n.d.; Lourens, 2024).

In 2022, the government enacted the 'Health Futures Act' to ensure that everyone could access quality healthcare. A key component of this reform was the centralisation of the previously fragmented healthcare system. This led to the dissolution of the 20 District Health Boards and the creation of Te Whatu Ora – Health New Zealand, a unified organisation. Additionally, the government established the 'Māori Health Authority,' with spending power, to ensure the Māori community is involved at every level of decision-making (Ministry of Health, 2023).

By mid-2024, these reforms were fully implemented, with both organisations fully operational.

Health New Zealand is the national health agency responsible for delivering healthcare services across the country. It oversees the daily operations of the country's healthcare system through four regional divisions. These work with district offices to develop and implement plans tailored to local community needs.

The Agency is responsible for the management of all healthcare services, encompassing hospital, primary, and community care. National planning of hospitals and specialised services aims to ensure consistent delivery throughout the country, and the organisation also oversees national contracts (Health New Zealand, 2021).

According to the most recent data from 2011, health insurance covers the entire population of New Zealand. This coverage encompasses both those who are members of health insurance schemes and those who have free access to state-provided healthcare services (Our World in Data, n.p.).

Public vs private

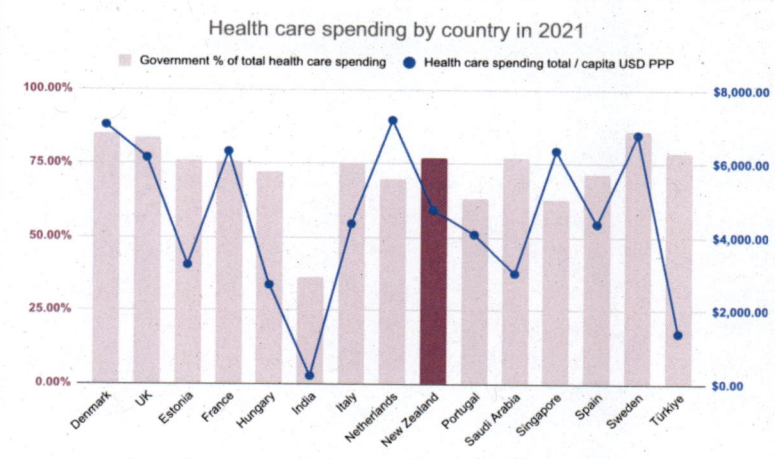

Figure 161. Source: The World Bank. The pink column refers to the public expenditure as a % of the country's total healthcare expenditure. The blue dot is the country's expenditure on health per capita, expressed in international dollars at purchasing power parity.

The national infrastructure

My Health Account is a digital health identity service provided by Health New Zealand. It allows individuals aged 16 and over to securely access online health services from anywhere. This service helps users verify their identity digitally, ensuring that only they can view and manage their personal health data. By creating a My Health Account, users can confidently access and control their health information, deciding when and with whom to share it. Additionally, parents can manage important health information for their children by linking their accounts (Te Whatu Ora, n.d.).

Portals

There is currently no national government portal or personal health records platform in New Zealand. Instead, the market comprises three privately owned GP portal systems. Through one of these platforms, Manage My Health, patients can also receive their hospital care documents.

To access their primary care information, patients can inquire at the reception of their GP or another community healthcare provider about registering for the patient portal they use. Once registered, patients can access certain health information, depending on the features offered by the portal. For example, they may be able to view:

- Health conditions
- Allergies
- Prescriptions
- Immunisations
- Lab results
- Clinician notes
- Upcoming appointments
- Hospital clinic letters, discharge summaries, and referral updates (via the Manage My Health portal)

Some portals also allow patients to interact with healthcare providers through features such as:

- Appointment booking
- Requesting repeat prescriptions
- Messaging their GP

Patients should check with their healthcare provider to find out which functions are available. The portals currently in use are (Ministry of Health, New Zealand Government, n.d.):

- [Manage My Health](): the platform used by most GP practices in New Zealand, developed in 2008 and now partnered with Health New Zealand
- [Health 365](): a platform used by some GPs
- [ConnectMed](): owned by Cereus

Bibliography

- Givealittle, n.d. St John National. Available at: [https://givealittle.co.nz/org/stjohnnational]() (accessed: 24 July 2024).

- Health New Zealand, 2021. Our health and disability system. Available at: [https://www.dpmc.govt.nz/sites/default/files/2021-04/htu-factsheet-health-new-zealand-en-apr21.pdf]() (accessed: 24 July 2024).

- Lourens, M., 2024. 'Part-funded paramedics: Should our ambulance service be government-run?', The Press, 16 February. Available at: [https://www.thepress.co.nz/nz-news/350172288/part-funded-paramedics-should-our-ambulance-service-be-government-run]() (accessed: 24 July 2024).

- Ministry of Health, 2022. Pae Ora (Healthy Futures) Act 2022. Available at: [https://legislation.govt.nz/act/public/2022/0030/latest/LMS575405.html]() (accessed: 24 July 2024).

- Ministry of Health, 2023. Health system reforms. Available at: [https://www.health.govt.nz/new-zealand-health-system/health-system-reforms]() (accessed: 24 July 2024).

- Ministry of Health, New Zealand Government., n.d. Te Whatu Ora - Health New Zealand - Access your healthcare information. Accessed at: [https://www.northlanddhb.org.nz/your-health/patient-and-visitor-information/access-your-healthcare-information/]() (accessed: 25 January 2024).

- PHARMAC, n.d. Home. Available at: [https://pharmac.govt.nz/]() (accessed: 24 July 2024).

- Scoop Health Independent News. Hospital Manage My Health Launched Today, 29 March 2023. Accessed at: [https://www.scoop.co.nz/stories/GE2303/S00073/hospital-]()

manage-my-health-launched-today.htm (accessed: 25 January 2024).

- Southern Health, n.d. About the New Zealand Health Care System. Available at: https://www.southernhealth.nz/getting-help-you-need/how-health-system-works/about-new-zealand-health-care-system (accessed: 24 July 2024).

- Te Whatu Ora, n.d. My Health Account. Available at: https://identity.health.nz/ (accessed: 24 July 2024).

- Te Whatu Ora, n.d. About My Health Account. Available at: https://www.tewhatuora.govt.nz/health-services-and-programmes/digital-health/my-health-account/about/ (accessed: 24 July 2024).

- Te Whatu Ora, n.d. Home. Available at: https://www.tewhatuora.govt.nz/ (accessed: 24 July 2024).

- Te Whatu Ora, n.d. Māori Health. Available at: https://www.tewhatuora.govt.nz/health-services-and-programmes/maori-health/ (accessed: 24 July 2024).

NEW ZEALAND – MANAGE MY HEALTH

History

Manage My Health was developed in 2008 by Medtech Global, a New Zealand-based company specialised in healthcare technology solutions. This patient portal can be integrated with various Electronic Health Records (EHR) systems and is used by most GP practices across the country, making it the most widely used patient portal in New Zealand. In 2020, when Cereus Holdings sold Medtech Global, it decided to retain ownership of the Manage My Health platform, continuing to operate it independently (Manage My Health, 2024,-a; McDonald, 2020).

Features

The platform grants patients access to their medical records from the Patient Management System of their registered practice. Registration starts through the website: Connect with your GPs with Manage My Health.

Manage My Health receives health information directly from a patient's doctor. Additionally, patients can manually enter details not recorded in the doctor's system, such as alternative treatments and medications. Currently, patients can access their health records through the portal, which includes recent medical conditions, immunisation records, allergies, prescriptions, and more. Furthermore, patients can:

- Book appointments with their GP
- Make online real-time payments for video and phone consultations, appointments, and repeat prescriptions
- Access lab test results as soon as their doctor receives them
- Order repeat prescriptions
- Receive appointment reminders
- Set and manage health goals
- Participate in video and phone consultations
- Send messages to doctors and nurses
- Share health information with healthcare providers and trusted individuals in case of emergencies

The website also offers non-record features, including access to health-related news, participation in community forums, and entry into various wellness initiatives (Manage My Health, 2024).

Challenges and areas for improvement

Manage My Health is widely used but faces several challenges that affect its functionality and user experience (PKB interviews, 2024). Key issues include:

- **Limited Data Integration**: The platform only aggregates information from GP practices and public healthcare providers, excluding data from private healthcare providers.
- **Lack of Access Log**: Patients cannot view an access log to see who has accessed their medical records or when limiting transparency.
- **Device Integration**: The platform does not currently support integration with health-monitoring devices, restricting its utility for patients who use such tools to manage their health.

Published outcomes - statistics

Manage My Health is used by over 1.85 million people (out of a total of 5.123 million population of New Zealand) and by most GP practices (Manage My Health, 2024,-b).

Screenshots

Screenshots are available on our website, phrs4govs.org.

The homepage provides patients with access to various sections of the portal. Key sections include the option to book an appointment with their GP, request a new repeat prescription, and view their health records, lab results, and messages from their healthcare provider, as well as the name of their GP health centre. Additionally, patients can click to access their 'health indicators' and review their health documents.

On the 'Schedule Your Appointment Now' page, patients can book an appointment by selecting or typing the reason for their visit. They can choose their preferred healthcare provider from their health centre and specify whether the appointment should be conducted in person or online.

In the 'My Health Record' section, patients can access an overview of their health information, which includes summaries, prescriptions, lab results, conditions, allergies, immunisations, clinical notes, and recalls. Within the summary section, patients can view their 'Health Summary' and download it as a PDF if needed. This summary contains information including the patient's demographics, recent healthcare encounters, current medications, allergies, significant health issues (such as smoking status), immunisations, diagnostic results, and vital signs.

On the 'Prescriptions' page, patients can view entries from their health centre and add their medications. For each entry, patients can see the date the prescription was issued, the name of the medication, detailed instructions for use, and the name of the prescribing healthcare provider.

Patients can add details about the medications they have taken, including the name of the medication, the quantity consumed, and the dosage. Additionally, they can specify the frequency of administration, the current status (indicating whether they are still taking the medication or not), and the relevant dates associated with each entry.

On the 'Conditions' page, patients can view the health conditions recorded by their health centre as well as those they have entered themselves. For each condition, patients can see the date it was recorded and the type of condition.

On the 'Lab Results' page, patients can view a list of their test results, accompanied by comments from their clinician. Each entry includes the health centre where the tests were performed and the date the results were received.

When patients click on a specific result, they can view detailed information pertaining to that test. Results are not presented in grouped formats or graphs; each result is displayed individually.

In the 'Clinician Notes' section, patients can access records of their visits, including the date of each appointment, the type of consultation, the name of the clinician, the health centre where the appointment took place, and the notes taken during the visit. Additionally, patients have the option to add their notes from other appointments.

In the 'Recalls' section, each entry includes the due date for the recall, a brief description of the procedure or action required, the recall code, and any associated letters.

Bibliography

- Manage My Health, 2024, My Health in My Hands. Available at: https://managemyhealth.co.nz/individuals/ (accessed: 25 January 2024).

- Manage My Health, 2024, About Us. Manage My Health. Available at: https://managemyhealth.co.nz/about-us/ (accessed: 25 July 2024).

- McDonald, K., 2020. Private equity firm buys Medtech Global, ManageMyHealth spun out. Pulse+IT News. Available at: https://www.pulseit.news/new-zealand-digital-health/private-equity-firm-buys-medtech-global-managemyhealth-spun-out/ (accessed: 25 July 2024).

PORTUGAL

Portugal was the first country in Europe to decriminalize the possession and use of all drugs in 2001. Since then, drug-related deaths have remained below the European Union average; the proportion of prisoners sentenced for drug offenses has decreased from 40% to 15%; and rates of drug use have consistently been below the EU average (Transform Drug Policy Foundation 2021).

Country's healthcare system in a nutshell

Portugal has universal health coverage through its public healthcare system, known as the Serviço Nacional de Saúde (SNS). The government is both the payer and the provider. As a provider, the SNS operates and manages healthcare facilities, including hospitals, health centres, and clinics, and employs a substantial portion of the healthcare workforce. As a payer, the government finances the SNS through public funds, covering healthcare costs and managing subsidies and co-payments to ensure access to care for all citizens and legal residents of Portugal. National health coverage includes all medical care, with the exception of dental care costs (Global Citizen Solutions, 2024).

Co-payments are only required for emergency services if the patient is not referred by the SNS or if hospitalisation does not occur. This is under Law Decree No. 37/2022. Where co-payments are applicable, exemptions exist for those experiencing financial hardship and for certain groups. These exempt groups include pregnant women; women in labour; children under 13 years old; individuals with a disability of 60% or more; blood donors; living donors of cells, tissues, and organs; firefighters; transplant patients; and military or former military personnel who are permanently disabled due to service (SNS24, 2022).

Health insurance covers the entire population of Portugal, according to the most recent data from 2010. This coverage encompasses both those who are members of health insurance schemes and those who have free access to state-provided healthcare services (Our World in Data, n.p.).

Public vs private

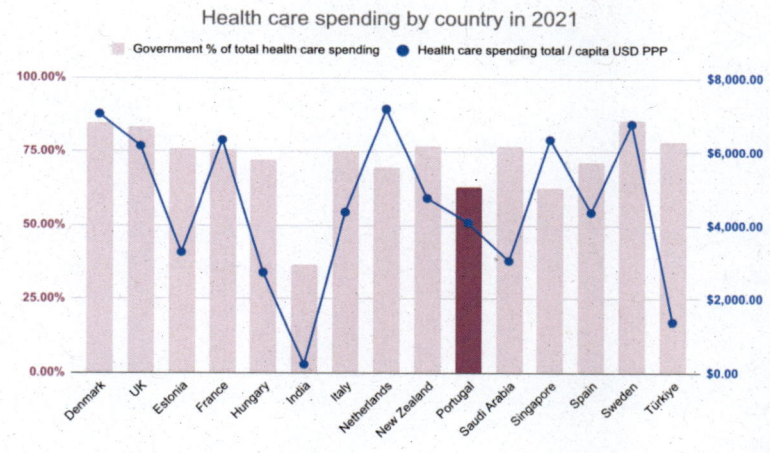

Figure 162. Source: The World Bank. The pink column refers to the public expenditure as a % of the country's total healthcare expenditure. The blue dot is the country's expenditure on health per capita, expressed in international dollars at purchasing power parity.

The national PHR

History

Over the years, Portugal developed various digital healthcare platforms for different purposes. The first patient-facing system, created in 2008/9, was an e-booking platform for individuals to schedule appointments with their GPs. The second portal, launched in 2011, enabled patients to check their waiting times for surgery (PKB interviews, 2023).

It was not until 2011, during the country's financial crisis – when Portugal required a bailout – that the first steps towards a more comprehensive patient portal were taken. As part of the EU Commission's conditions for granting a €75 billion loan, Portugal was given 11 months to create a platform for data sharing called the Personal Computer Record (PKB interviews, 2023).

Henrique Martins, at the time president of Portugal's Digital Health Agency (SPMS), proposed the creation of three portals: a professional, a patient, and an institutional one.

The patient portal launched first (April 2012), followed by the professional portal (July 2012), which connected 365 health centres. An accompanying app was introduced in 2017.

The development and implementation of the platform faced several challenges. Most notably, the project initially had a very low budget of €60,000, as it was difficult to gain political recognition of the economic value of patient empowerment. However, the situation improved the following year, and by 2023, total investment in the portal had reached €5–6 million. Another significant challenge was the shortage of programming skills among the population (PKB interviews, 2023).

Public portal (SNS 24)

SNS 24, operated by the Portuguese National Health Service, functions through four channels: the SNS 24 Portal, Telephone Line, SNS 24 App, and SNS 24 Counter. Each channel is dedicated to delivering information and services to citizens, enhancing the accessibility of the National Health Service (SNS) to the public (SNS24 website, 2024).

Within the platform, the electronic health record (EHR) portal, SNS 24 Portal, consists of two areas: the citizen area and the professional area. The professional area supports clinical procedures, allowing healthcare professionals working within the SNS to access EHR data from different healthcare facilities, including primary care units and tertiary care units (SNS24 website, 2024).

Citizens can log into their 'personal area' on the SNS 24 Portal, where they can access the following health information collected at SNS institutions:

- Their identification and contact details
- The health centre where they are registered
- Benefits granted, such as exemptions and contributions
- Allergies
- Current medications
- Diagnoses and conditions
- Their position on the surgery waiting list, if applicable
- Vaccination record
- Habits, such as alcohol consumption
- Test results/measurements: BMI, Glycaemia, Blood pressure, Triglycerides, O2 saturation, INR, Heart rate, Total cholesterol, LDL cholesterol, HDL cholesterol, HbA1c
- Organ donor status

Patients can also add their own data to most of the fields listed above, but they must choose from predefined options. For instance, they cannot manually enter a condition but must choose from a drop-down menu of conditions. Users can choose who can access their information, such as GPs or hospital doctors.

At launch, the platform only collected data from public providers and GPs. Over time, some private healthcare providers joined SNS 24, while others continued to use different platforms. Certain types of patient data, such as prescriptions, sick leave, and certificates (e.g., doctor's certificates for driving licences), are present in the SNS 24 portal regardless of the provider.

There are two different rules for data access:

- All professionals can access all data entered by any healthcare professional, whether from a private or public provider.
- Professionals can only access data the patient entered if the patient lets them.

Public app SNS24

Through the SNS24 App, patients can access the following services:

- Vaccination Bulletin
- Declaration of contact with the SNS 24 Line
- Sick leave
- Treatment Guides and dispensed medication leaflets
- Health Agenda
- Self-Declaration of Illness
- ADSE Card
- Blood donor card
- Living will
- Multipurpose Disability Medical Certificate
- QR Code – Electronic Kiosk
- Pathologies (allergies and rare diseases)
- Exams (Performance and Results Guide)
- Clinical referrals
- Consultation of usual medication
- Application for renewal of usual medication
- Contacts of health facilities
- Contact with SNS 24 – via 808242424 and using the accessible contact (Portuguese Sign Language)

- Teleconsultation (via CSR Live)
- Availability for teleconsultation: the user registers his/her availability to make teleconsultation
- EU Digital COVID Certificate
- Possibility to add multiple users
- Access to the SNS 24 portal
- Access to the App MySNS
- Access to the App MySNS Times
- Access to the App Telemonit SNS 24
- Record 3 types of measurements: Glycaemia, Blood pressure, Body Mass Index

Comparison Between SNS24 Portal and App

Features	Portal	App
Surgical waiting list, organ donor status, habits tracking, and control over provider access to health data.	Yes	No
Appointment management, teleconsultation, and clinical referrals.	No	Yes

Challenges and areas for improvement

Several challenges were encountered during the development and implementation of the system:

- The private healthcare sector's formal agreement or strategy was never developed. As a result, the platform's data is limited to contributions from public healthcare providers, with some exceptions. This may be a key reason why patient usage growth has been steady but never exponential.

- Low digital literacy among patients. 20% of the Portuguese population has never used the internet. To overcome this challenge, since 2015, administrative staff have been assisting patients in navigating the portal.

The primary weaknesses are the lack of data from most private healthcare providers and the inability to integrate with medical devices. Moreover, although patients can add personal data to their records, they are limited to selecting from pre-defined options, such as choosing from a drop-down menu of diseases. Additionally, patients are unable to share their records with trustees (PKB interviews, 2023).

Screenshots

Screenshots are available on our website, phrs4govs.org.

Homepage

The home page features links to four main areas.

'My Area' (top left): essential personal information, including identification details, emergency contacts, advance directives, authorisations, and a log of who has accessed their information.

'I Need To...' (top right): allows various actions. A person can book a consultation for themselves or others, request a referral, check their test results and medical leave, see details about upcoming surgeries, access home respiratory care, obtain proof of attendance, get their COVID digital certificate, and consult attestations or self-declarations of illness.

'My Records' (bottom left): shows the health summary, medical reports, diabetes risk calculator, and patient measurements. Patients can also review health data they have personally entered, individual care plans, their rare diseases card, and their non-donor status.

'Know More' (bottom right): provides information on co-payments, treatments abroad, a list of healthcare providers, and a library of informative resources.

Data from the patient

Measurements

In the 'measurements' area, patients can self-enter their measurements.

Patients can add various health measurements to their records, but only those provided in the platform's predefined list. The available measurements include Body Mass Index (BMI), glycemia, blood pressure, triglycerides, oxygen saturation (O_2 saturation), International Normalised Ratio (INR), heart rate, total cholesterol, LDL cholesterol, HDL cholesterol, and HbA1c.

Habits

In the 'My Habits' section, patients have the opportunity to log and monitor their lifestyle choices. This includes recording their eating habits, indicating whether they smoke, detailing their alcohol consumption, and noting any sports or physical activities they engage in.

Medications

Patients can self-enter the medications they are currently taking. This feature allows them to select their medicines from a dropdown list, specify the start date and duration of the treatment, and provide an explanation of the reason for each medication.

Allergies

Patients can document any allergies in their health records. This includes specifying the date of the allergy, identifying the allergen, detailing the reaction experienced, assessing the severity of the reaction, and providing any additional descriptions or observations.

Conditions

Patients can include any medical conditions or diagnoses in their health records. This feature allows them to specify the date the condition began, the date it ended (if applicable), and any additional comments or observations.

Certificates

Rare disease card

In their health records, patients can view their rare disease card if they have been diagnosed with a rare disease. This feature is particularly valuable for emergency care, as it provides critical information about the patient's condition, ensuring that healthcare providers can respond appropriately in urgent situations.

Non-donation

The non-donor individual card is designed for those who choose not to be organ donors, as Portuguese law automatically designates individuals as donors at birth.

Bibliography

- AMA Administrative Modernization Agency. (n.d) Consult the personal area of the SNS 24 portal. Available at: https://www2.gov.pt/en-GB/servicos/consultar-o-meu-registo-de-saude-eletronico (accessed: 7 September 2023).

- SNS24, 2022. End of user fees in the NHS (online) 1 June. Available at: https://www.sns.gov.pt/noticias/2022/06/01/fim-das-taxas-moderadoras-no-sns-2/ (accessed: 24 July 2024).

- SNS24, 2024. About Us. Available at: https://www.sns24.gov.pt/how-can-sns24-help-me/ (accessed: 1 May 2024).

- SNS24, 2024. SNS24 App. Available at: https://www.sns24.gov.pt/sobre-nos/ (accessed: 1 May 2024).

- Teixeira, J.G., de Pinho, N.F. and Patrício, L., 2019. Bringing service design to the development of health information systems: The case of the Portuguese national electronic health record. International journal of medical informatics, 132, p.103942. Available at: https://doi.org/10.1016/j.ijmedinf.2019.08.002 (accessed: 3 November 2024).

- Leontina Postelnicu, 2020. How Portugal is advancing the use of eHealth in Europe. Available at: https://www.healthcareit-news.com/news/emea/how-portugal-advancing-use-ehealth-europe (accessed: 7 September 2023).

- Global Citizen Solutions. (Last updated 29 April 2024). The Portugal Healthcare System: a Guide for Expats. Available at: https://www.globalcitizensolutions.com/portugal-healthcare-foreigners/ (accessed: 1 May 2024).

- Transform Drug Policy Foundation 2021. Drug decriminalisation in Portugal: setting the record straight. Available at: https://transformdrugs.org/blog/drug-decriminalisation-in-portugal-setting-the-record-straight (accessed: 2 November 2024).

SAUDI ARABIA

Forty-two conjoined twins have been successfully separated by Saudi Arabia's former Minister of Health (Al Rabeeh 2009). The paediatric surgeon, Abdullah bin Abdulaziz Al Rabeeah, leads a team at the King Faisal Specialist Hospital and Research Centre, specialising in these cases from all over the world. This is one example of the Kingdom's investment in excellence.

Country's healthcare system in a nutshell

Saudi Arabia introduced universal health coverage in 2019 to ensure that both citizens and residents can access healthcare at no cost. Funding for the Ministry of Health primarily derives from the annual government budget, which is largely supported by oil revenues (Almodhen and Moneir, 2023).

Primary care is offered through primary healthcare centres (PHCs), which deliver essential services such as preventive care, health education, and screening. Secondary care is provided by hospitals and specialised centres that offer more advanced services, including diagnostic procedures, surgical operations, and emergency care. The most complex treatments are handled at tertiary care hospitals, specialising in areas such as organ transplants and cancer therapy.

Despite significant improvements, the system faces ongoing challenges, including a shortage of healthcare professionals, insufficient preventive care, and notable disparities in healthcare access between urban and rural regions (Gurajala, 2023).

To address these issues, the Saudi government launched the 'Vision 2030' initiative, aimed at enhancing public services across various sectors, including healthcare. As part of the initiative, in 2022, the Ministry of Health established the Health Holding Company (HHC), a state-owned enterprise designed to transform the nation's healthcare system. The HHC's mandate includes taking over the provision of healthcare services, while the Ministry's role shifts from service provision to supervision and regulation.

The HHC is leading several key reforms, including (Ministry of Health, 2022):

- **Decentralisation**: the HHC is responsible for creating and delegating the delivery of healthcare services to 20 regional clusters to encourage local involvement and improve responsiveness to community needs.
- **Privatisation**: the HHC will privatise numerous public hospitals and primary health centres.
- **Digitisation**: the strategy includes a push towards digital healthcare, enhancing data interoperability, and expanding access to digital and virtual medical services. This is particularly crucial for the roughly 16% of the population living in remote areas with limited access to healthcare services.
- **Specialised Care Services**: the HHC will offer specialised services such as cancer care, renal rehabilitation, and critical care in cardiology and trauma. A new Model of Care, encompassing 42 interventions across six healthcare systems, aims to standardise and improve treatment based on evidence-based practices.
- **Community Health**: The HHC will also focus on disease prevention and early detection, aiming to improve community health across the country.
- **Workforce Development**: The transformation plan includes workforce planning and development, with an emphasis on improving training standards and ensuring an adequate supply of healthcare professionals to meet the country's growing needs.

Public vs private

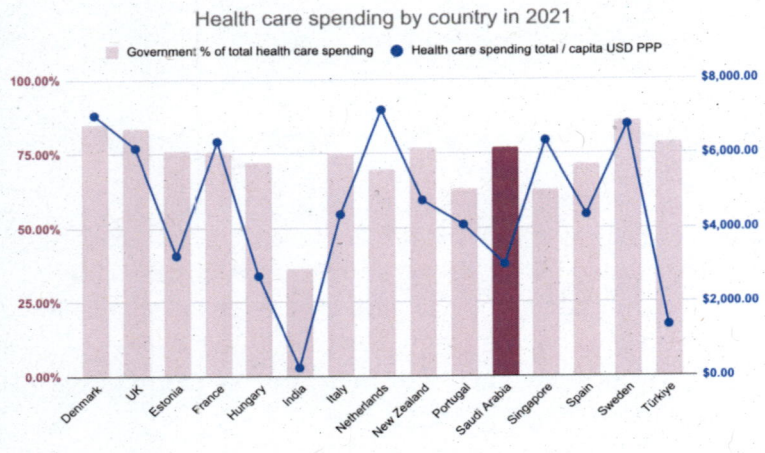

Figure 163. Source: The World Bank. The pink column refers to the public expenditure as a % of the country's total healthcare expenditure. The blue dot is the country's expenditure on health per capita, expressed in international dollars at purchasing power parity.

The national PHR

History

The Saudi Ministry of Health commissioned and launched the Sehhaty application in August 2019 to achieve a number of national goals that focus on healthy lifestyles. In February 2021, the app was updated to include COVID-19 vaccination appointment registration and test booking, expanding its role in the nation's pandemic response.

Lean Business Services developed Sehhaty as a state-owned enterprise (Ministry of Health, 2021).

Sehhaty became the national platform for individuals' healthcare needs following MoH's announcement on the 2nd of September 2022. The ministry revealed plans to integrate all government health bodies with Sehhaty, ensuring the app would serve as a comprehensive platform for delivering health services. This announcement coincided with the MoH signing a cooperation agreement with the Digital Government Authority (DGA), marking the merger of various health sector platforms into Sehhaty. The integration aimed to centralise health data sources, improve service quality, and ultimately enhance patient satisfaction (Joseph, 2022).

Features

The Sehhaty platform serves all residents of the Kingdom of Saudi Arabia, along with their dependents, including children, the elderly, and individuals with special needs. The app is available in both Arabic and English.

Key services provided by Sehhaty include (Ministry of Health, 2023):

- Immediate virtual consultations
- Booking and reviewing appointments
- Remote appointments
- Medication search
- Digital Health Wallet
- Viewing sick leave and medical reports
- Women's health services
- Dependents' services
- A dedicated primary care doctor for each family member (My Doctor)
- Records of children's vaccinations and appointments
- Monitoring vital signs (via the "Know Your Numbers" service)
- Step counting

- Maintaining a list of medications
- Educational content
- Booking COVID-19 screening and vaccination appointments
- Booking general vaccination appointments
- Early weather condition alerts for asthmatics

Challenges and areas for improvement

Sehhaty provides a comprehensive range of services but has some limitations that affect its overall functionality (PKB interviews, 2024):

- **Lack of access Log**: Users cannot view an access log to track who has accessed their medical records or when, reducing transparency.
- **Closed platform**: Sehhaty does not integrate with third-party software, restricting its ability to work seamlessly with other health-related apps and systems.

Published outcomes - statistics

Unfortunately, we couldn't find any statistics about the use of Sehhaty in Saudi Arabia. If you have access to this information or can put us in touch with someone who has, please contact us at book@phr4gov.org.

Screenshots

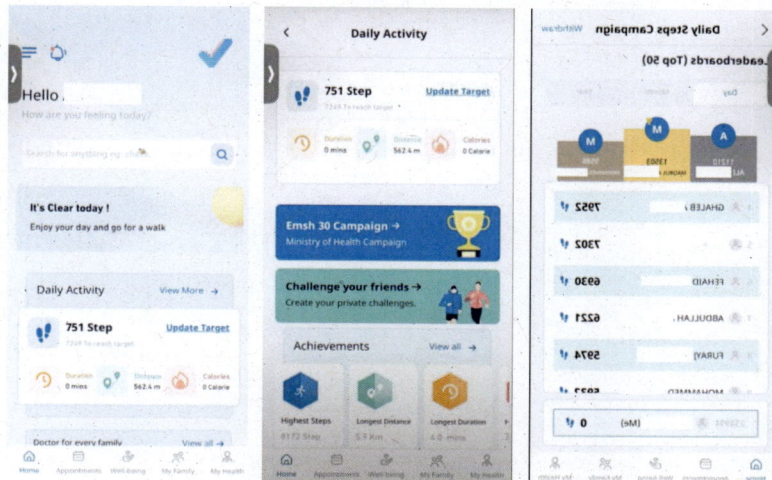

Figure 164. Home page: search function for patients to search for their data; weather, which, in case of an allergic person, will suggest whether to go out or not based on pollen; step count that takes information directly from the mobile phone.

Figure 165. Home page, gamification part related to steps.

Figure 166. Home page, gamification part related to steps.

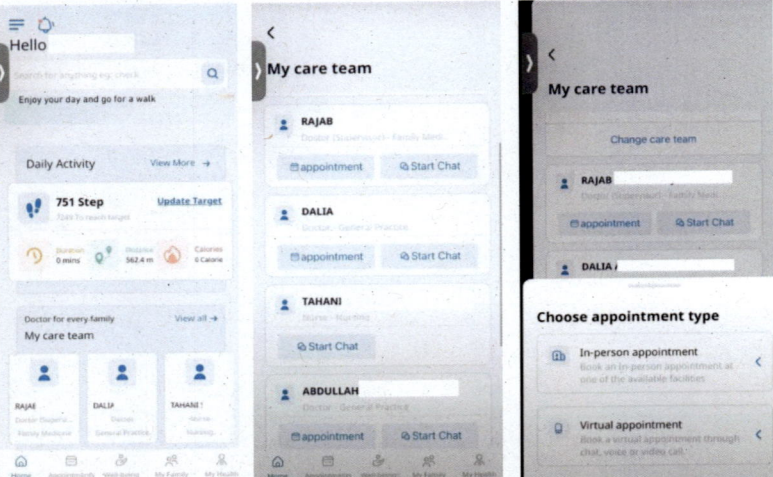

Figure 167. My care team: here, patients can see their healthcare professionals.

Figure 168. View when patients open the 'My care team' tab.

Figure 169. Once patients open the list of professionals, they can book an appointment with one of them (in person or virtual).

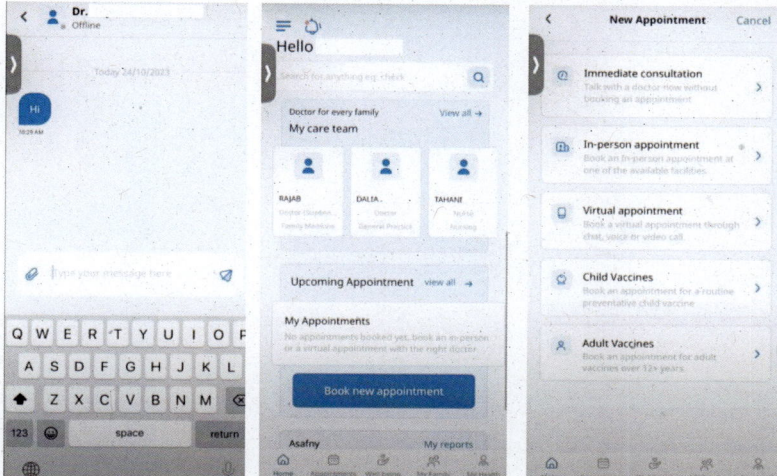

Figure 170. Patients can also click on a professional and send him/her a message.

Figure 171. On the homepage, patients can also see their upcoming appointment or book a new one.

Figure 172. This is the view once the patient clicks on 'book new appointment.'

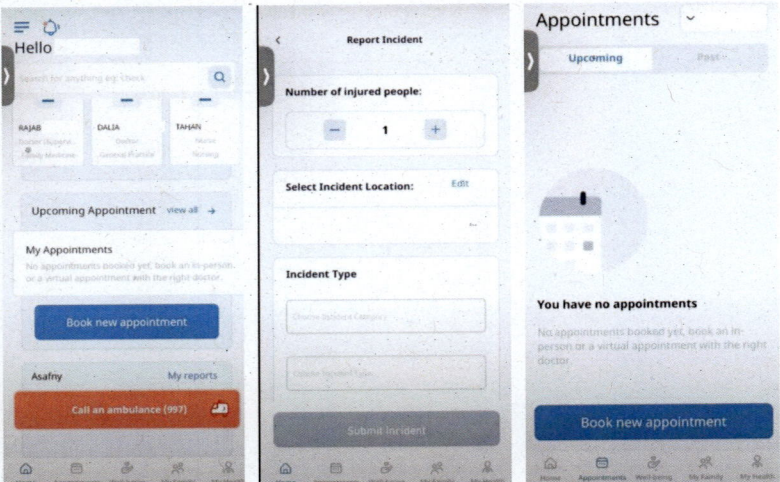

Figure 173. On the homepage, patients have the option to call an ambulance.

Figure 174. The call ambulance feature sends the position automatically. Patients can add the type of incident and the number of people injured.

Figure 175. Next to the homepage is the appointments tab. Here, patients can see past and upcoming appointments and book new ones.

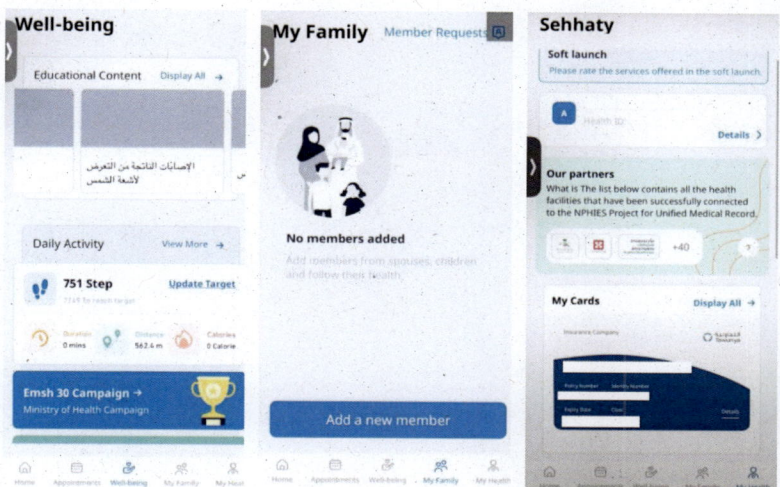

Figure 176. In the Well-being tab, patients can find a library of educational resources for their conditions and the steps count.

Figure 177. In the 'My Family' tab, patients can add people they look after by sending them a request to access their records. These can be spouses, children, or others.

Figure 178. In the 'My Health' tab, patients can see the list of health facilities that are connected to the Sahhaty platform and their insurance health card.

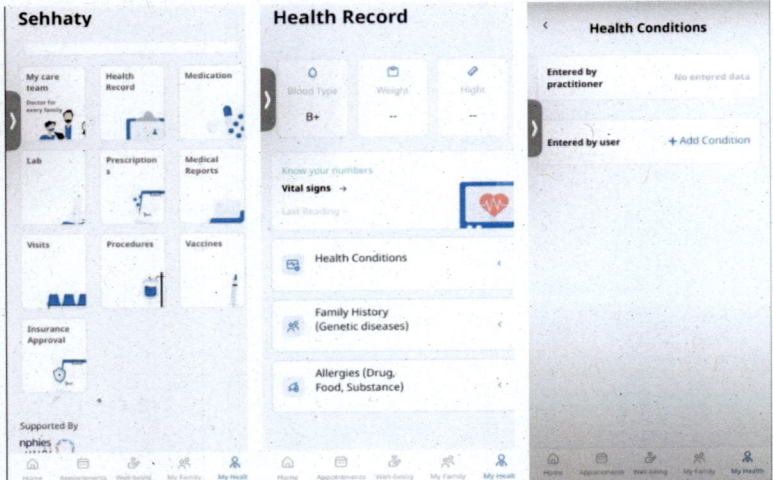

Figure 179. Scrolling down in the 'My Health' tab, patients can see their doctors, their health record, their medications, lab results, prescriptions, medical reports, visits, procedures, vaccines, and insurance approval.

Figure 180. Within the 'health record,' patients can see and add their blood type, their weight and height, their conditions, family history, and allergies.

Figure 181. Data can be added by a professional or by patients themselves.

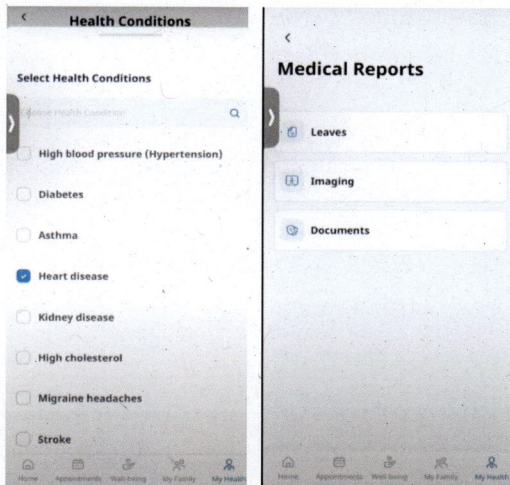

Figure 182. For example, patients can select their conditions from a list.

Figure 183. Within 'Medical Reports,' patients can see their leaves, imaging results (the report but not the imaging itself), and documents.

Bibliography

- Almodhen, F. and Moneir, W.M., 2023. Toward a Financially Sustainable Healthcare System in Saudi Arabia. Cureus, 15(10). Available at: https://www.ncbi.nlm.nih.gov/pmc/articles/PMC10632744/ (accessed: 2 November 2024).

- Alqahtani, W.S., Almufareh, N.A., Domiaty, D.M., Albasher, G., Alduwish, M.A., Alkhalaf, H., Almuzzaini, B., Al-Marshidy, S.S., Alfraihi, R., Elasbali, A.M. and Ahmed, H.G., 2020. Epidemiology of cancer in Saudi Arabia thru 2010–2019: a systematic review with constrained meta-analysis. AIMS Public Health, 7(3), p.679. Available at: https://pmc.ncbi.nlm.nih.gov/articles/PMC7505779/ (accessed: 2 November 2024).

- Al Rabeeah, A.A., 2009. My experience with the conjoined twins (Arabic). Riyadh: Al Obeikan Co., Research and Development. Print.

- Dawood, A. M., & Alkadi, K. S., 2022. Evaluating Usability of Telehealth Sehhaty Application Used in Saudi Arabia During Covid-19. Studies in health technology and informatics, 295, 285–288. Available at: https://ebooks.iospress.nl/doi/10.3233/SHTI220718 (accessed: 3 November 2024).

- Gurajala, S., 2023. Healthcare System in the Kingdom of Saudi Arabia: An Expat Doctor's Perspective. Cureus, 15(5). Available at: https://www.ncbi.nlm.nih.gov/pmc/articles/PMC10250784/ (accessed: 2 November 2024).

- Joseph, S. A., 2022. Saudi Arabia picks Sehhaty app as national e-platform for healthcare services. GCC Business News. Available at: https://www.gccbusinessnews.com/saudi-arabia-picks-sehhaty-app-as-national-e-platform-for-healthcare-services/ (accessed: 1 November 2023).

- Ministry of Health, 2021. Partnership Agreement with 'Lean.' Available at: https://www.moh.gov.sa/en/Ministry/Partnerships/Pages/Lean-Company.aspx (accessed: 1 November 2023).

- Ministry of Health, 2023. "Sehhaty" Platform. Available at: https://www.moh.gov.sa/en/eServices/Sehhaty/Pages/default.aspx (accessed: 1 November 2023).

- Ministry of Health, n.d. Health Sector Transformation Strategy, Vision 2030. Available at: https://www.moh.gov.sa/en/Ministry/vro/Documents/Healthcare-Transformation-Strategy.pdf (accessed: 1 August 2024).

SINGAPORE

Singapore's spending on health care is lower than that of every OECD country. It is just 5.6% of GDP. Yet Singapore's health outcomes are better than those of most prosperous countries. Its government does this by focusing on the causes of good health, such as diet, exercise, and screening. The government also reduces the price of health care by forcing direct payments (instead of insurance) and by strict cost controls (without rationing).

Country's healthcare system in a nutshell

The healthcare system in Singapore is managed by the Ministry of Health, which is part of the Singaporean government. The country has achieved universal health coverage through a mixed financing system known as the 3Ms: MediShield Life, MediSave, and Medi-Fund. These schemes can overlap to cover the costs of a single treatment episode.

MediShield Life is a mandatory universal insurance scheme for citizens and permanent residents. It covers large hospital bills and certain costly outpatient treatments. However, it does not cover primary care, outpatient specialist consultations, and prescription medications. For these, patients must pay premiums, deductibles, co-insurance, and any costs that exceed claim limits. MediShield Life is complemented by MediSave, a compulsory medical savings account that helps residents cover inpatient and selected outpatient costs, including out-of-pocket expenses. Contributions to MediSave, which range from 8% to 10.5% of an individual's salary depending on age, are mandatory for all working citizens and permanent residents. Separately, residents may choose to purchase supplementary private insurance or receive employer-provided coverage. MediFund is a safety net the government provides. It is for low-income individuals who cannot afford healthcare costs, even with MediSave (Tikkanen et al., 2020).

According to the most recent data from 2010, health insurance covers the entire population of Singapore. This coverage encompasses both those who are members of health insurance schemes and those who have free access to state-provided healthcare services (Our World in Data, n.p.).

Global consulting firm Towers Watson has recognized Singapore as having "one of the most successful healthcare systems in the world, in terms of both efficiency in financing and the results achieved in community health outcomes" (Tucci, 2004).

Demand for senior care will significantly rise as the number of elderly citizens in Singapore reaches 900,000 by 2030 and birth rates are low. This makes healthcare needs a top priority, according to the 'Smart Nation Singapore' webpage. As part of its Smart Nation initiative, Singapore continues to explore technological solutions to meet these evolving healthcare needs.

Currently, health initiatives focus on equipping Singaporeans with the information and tools to manage their health more effectively. One such initiative is HealthHub.

Public vs private

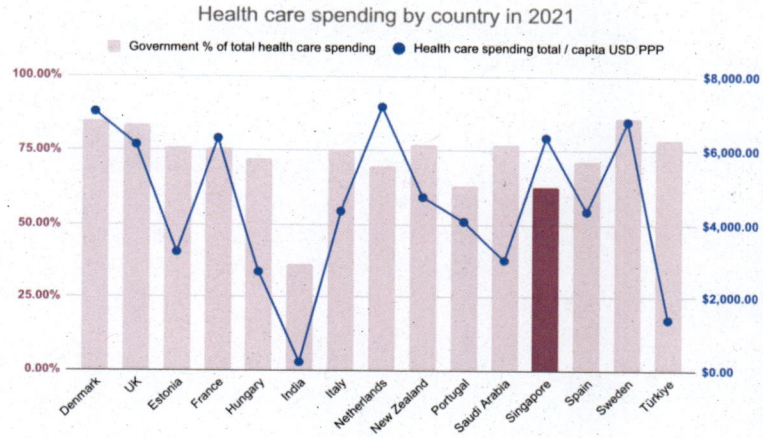

Figure 184. Source: The World Bank. The pink column refers to the public expenditure as a % of the country's total healthcare expenditure. The blue dot is the country's expenditure on health per capita, expressed in international dollars at purchasing power parity.

The national PHR

History

To understand Singapore's national Personal Health Record, we must begin with the National Electronic Health Record (NEHR).

All public and private healthcare institutions have implemented NEHR since 2011. It is a fundamental component of the country's vision of 'One Patient, One Health Record,' so patients receive coordinated, patient-centred care. Authorised clinicians and healthcare professionals—including doctors, nurses, and pharmacists—have secure access to a patient's summary health record.

This promotes better care coordination and informed decision-making and supports accurate diagnosis and treatment.

The data in NEHR focuses on a summary of the patient's medical history rather than detailed doctors' notes for each consultation. The summary health records are transmitted from providers' electronic systems to the NEHR. NEHR's data requirements include patient demographics, patient visits, diagnoses, discharge summaries, medications, laboratory reports, radiology images and reports, notes, procedures, treatments, immunizations, allergies, referral notes, appointments, problem lists, ECGs, and care management programs (care plans).

The NEHR is owned by the Ministry of Health and managed by Synapxe (formerly known as the Integrated Health Information Systems, IHiS), an organisation established by the Ministry of Health.

Patients do not have direct access to the NEHR itself. However, they can see some of their clinical records held within the NEHR through the government portal 'HealthHub' (Synapxe Pte Ltd, 2024).

The concept for a comprehensive portal and mobile app providing Singaporeans with access to a variety of health content and e-services was first conceived in late 2013. HealthHub, an initiative by the Ministry of Health and the Health Promotion Board - with support from MOH Holdings and Integrated Health Information Systems (IHiS) - began development in May 2014. The portal launched in 2015, featuring both a web platform and a mobile application. It included a Personal Health Record function known as 'myHealth' (GovInsider, 2015; Government Technology Agency of Singapore, 2017).

Features

HealthHub shows information from various systems, including the NEHR, School Health System, School Dental System, and the National Immunisation Registry. It provides access to a wide range of data from public healthcare institutions, including (Synapxe Pte Ltd, 2024):

- Hospital records, such as hospital discharge summaries
- Lab test results (particularly for chronic diseases)
- Medical appointments
- Referral letters
- Immunisation records
- Dental health information
- Medication records, including prescriptions—patients can also set reminders for when to take their medication
- Screening records
- Risk assessments for diabetes
- Information on lifestyle facilities and services, such as the locations of polyclinics, healthy food outlets, and sports facilities

The Caregiver Access module allows a patient to grant carers access to their medical records and appointments. Parents are also able to access and add data to their children's health records.

Medical fee payments are also possible via the platform.

Challenges and areas for improvement

Data fragmentation was a challenge during the development of HealthHub. The platform needed to integrate data from various IT systems used by public hospitals and clinics before it could show the information unified (GovInsider, 2015).

While HealthHub offers valuable services, there are several areas for enhancement (PKB research, 2024):

- **Limited Data Entry**: Patients can only input limited personal data, specifically in the measurements section, while most of the record is 'view-only.'
- **Public sector**: The platform exclusively sources data from public institutions, limiting the comprehensiveness of the records.
- **Lack of Messaging Feature**: Patients cannot communicate directly with healthcare professionals through the platform.

Published outcomes - statistics

Unfortunately, we haven't found any recent statistics about the use of HealthHub in Singapore. If you have access to this information or can put us in touch with someone who has, please contact us at book@phr4gov.org

The latest available statistics are from January 2017, stating that the HealthHub website had 8.5 million page views and that over 84,000 Singaporeans had downloaded the app (Gov Tech Singapore website).

Screenshots

Screenshots are available on our website, phrs4govs.org.

Patients can log in to view and manage their medical records. Once logged in, they can access and manage their appointments, view vaccination records, and see test results from the past three years. Patients can also check medical alerts, adverse drug reactions, and allergies, as well as screening results and discharge and admission information from public hospitals or healthcare institutions (up to three years). Additionally, they can track measurements like blood glucose, blood pressure, and BMI, request certificates, view current prescriptions and medications, authorise the Ministry of Health for subsidies, MediSave, and MediShield Life, complete health-related self-assessments, make payments, request prescription renewals, check their Community Health Assist Scheme (CHAS) subsidy balance, see upcoming screenings, and view Chest X-Ray and Mammogram reports.

Citizens can use HealthHub to view and manage their children's records. This includes managing appointments, viewing allergies and adverse reactions, school referral and reminder letters, immunisation records, growth charts (from 0 to 18 years old), and developmental milestones (from 0 to 6 years old). Parents can also enter birth information, view the child's health assessment summary and dental records, access lab test results from the past three years, and see discharge and admission details. Additionally, parents can view radiology reports, authorise immunisation and preventive dental services, and apply for medical certificates.

Patients can use HealthHub to allow their caregivers access to their health records.

Bibliography

- GovInsider, 2015. How we built it... Singapore HealthHub. Available at: How we built it... Singapore HealthHub (accessed: 30 July 2024).

- Government Technology Agency of Singapore, 2017. A healthy hub at your fingertips. Available at: https://www.tech.gov.sg/media/technews/a-healthy-hub-at-your-fingertips/ (accessed: 30 July 2024).

- Smart Nation and Digital Government Office, 2024. Smart Health Initiatives. Available at: https://www.smartnation.gov.sg/initiatives/health/ (accessed: 30 July 2024).

- Synapxe Pte Ltd., 2024. About National Electronic Health Record (NEHR). Available at: NEHR (accessed: 30 July 2024).

- Tikkanen, R., Osborn, R., Mossialos, E., Djordjevic, A. and Wharton, G. A.,2020. International Health Care System Profiles, Singapore. The Commonwealth Fund. Available at: Singapore (accessed: 30 July 2024).

- Tucci, J. and Watson, T., 2004. The Singapore health system—achieving positive health outcomes with low expenditure. Healthcare Market Review, 26.

SPAIN

"Computers are useless.
They can only give you answers."

- Pablo Picasso, born in Andalucia, artist in Catalonia.

Country's healthcare system in a nutshell

38% of the European Union's high-speed rail track is in Spain (Eurostat, 2024). Spain's high-speed rail system is similar to its health care system. Both are decentralized but nationally integrated; efficient, fast, and cost-effective, focused on accessibility and equal opportunity.

Spain's National Health System (SNS) is predominantly funded through general taxation, providing universal access to a wide range of services for all residents, including citizens and documented and undocumented migrants (World Health Organization, 2023).

The Ministry of Health is responsible for national health planning and regulation. The 17 regional health authorities manage regional operational planning, resource allocation, and decisions regarding service provision. The SNS Interterritorial Council, which includes the national Minister of Health and the regional health ministers, coordinates high-level policies. Although there are minimal regional variations in coverage, there is variation in resource allocation.

Health services are delivered by a mix of public and private providers, with primary care doctors acting as gatekeepers to specialist and hospital care.

Each autonomous community, including Catalonia and Andalucia, has its own regional health authority responsible for managing and overseeing healthcare within its borders.

According to the most recent data from 2010, health insurance covered 99.2% of the population in Spain. This includes both those who are part of health insurance schemes and those who have free access to state-provided healthcare services (Our World in Data, n.p.).

Catalonia

The Generalitat de Catalonia governs Catalonia's healthcare system. This autonomous government enjoys a high degree of independence in healthcare decision-making. The Generalitat sets policies, allocates budgets, and administers healthcare services to meet the specific needs of its population. Additionally, Catalonia has developed its own digital health platform, La Meva Salut, which provides citizens with a range of services to access and manage their healthcare information (Dedeu, 2017).

Central government	Autonomous government of Catalonia
Basic legislation and coordination	Subsidiary legislation
Minimum package funded through NHS	Organisational structure of the health system
Pharmaceutical policy	Accreditation and planning
International health policy	Purchasing and service provision

Educational requirements	Public health
	Quality evaluation / Agency for Quality

Andalucia

Similarly, in Andalucía, the Junta de Andalucía holds significant authority over the region's healthcare system. The Junta is responsible for formulating healthcare policies, allocating budgets, and overseeing service provision within the region. Like Catalonia, Andalucía enjoys substantial independence in healthcare decision-making. The region has also developed its own digital health platform, ClicSalud+, which enables residents to access their health records and manage healthcare-related tasks online.

While both Catalonia and Andalucía have a high degree of autonomy in healthcare decision-making, the overarching framework of the Spanish healthcare system prioritises universal access and consistent standards. It ensures that residents across all regions receive a consistent level of quality care.

Public vs private

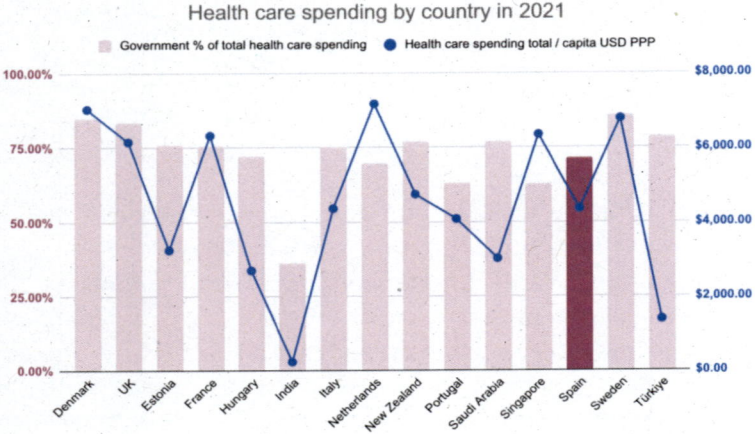

Figure 185. Source: The World Bank. The pink column refers to the public expenditure as a % of the country's total healthcare expenditure. The blue dot is the country's expenditure on health per capita, expressed in international dollars at purchasing power parity.

Bibliography

- Dedeu, T., 2017. *Health System Catalonia*. The presentation was given by Dr Toni Dedeu, Director General, Government of Catalonia, Ministry of Health, on 27 February. Available at: https://health.ec.europa.eu/system/files/2017-03/ev_20170227_co07_0.pdf (accessed: 30 July 2024).

- Eurostat, 2024. *Statistics Explained*. Available at: https://ec.europa.eu/eurostat/statistics-explained/index.php?oldid=631020 (accessed: 20 January 2025).

- World Health Organization, 2023. Spain: Country Health Profile 2023. State of Health in the EU. Available at: https://euro-healthobservatory.who.int/publications/m/spain-country-health-profile-2023 (accessed: 30 July 2024).

SPAIN – ANDALUCIA

History

ClicSalud+ serves as a virtual health management platform for residents with public health coverage in Andalusia, offering access to personal health information and the ability to manage appointments online (Servicio Andaluz de Salud, n.d). The platform ensures secure data transmission and user authentication through advanced technologies. It launched in 2002 (originally under the name InterSAS).

ClicSalud+ integrates with DIRAYA, the regional system consolidating all essential patient information into a unified profile. This profile - including administrative details, appointments, and clinical records - is accessible at any point of care, whether in an emergency room or hospital setting.

The integration of ClicSalud+ with these systems ensures that the data provided is up-to-date and that any user updates are promptly reflected across all associated information systems.

Access to these services requires user authentication. While some services can be accessed by providing personal details, others—due to their sensitive nature—require the use of a digital certificate.

Features

ClicSalud+ currently offers a range of features that enable patients to log in to access their health records, manage appointments, and request prescriptions. Features include (Servicio Andaluz de Salud, n.d):

- **Health agenda:**
  - ○ Request primary care appointments
  - ○ Reschedule or cancel certain types of upcoming appointments, as well as view a list of past ones
  - ○ Check position on the surgical waiting list
- **Health:**
  - ○ View information on medical conditions and allergies
  - ○ Access COVID-19 certificates
  - ○ Review medication and prescriptions
  - ○ Access clinical reports, such as admission records, hospitalisations, outpatient consultations, and discharge reports
  - ○ View analytical test results, such as blood tests
  - ○ Access imaging tests (note: patients can see the images, but not the clinician's written report)
  - ○ View vaccine records from 2010 onwards
  - ○ Check temporary disability information, particularly related to work incapacity
- **Formalities:**
  - ○ Request a new health card in the event of deterioration, loss, or theft
  - ○ Request a temporary displacement (e.g., if moving to a different Andalusian municipality, patients can choose a primary care centre and professional in the new location)
  - ○ Choose their GP

Challenges and areas for improvement

While **ClicSalud+** offers valuable services, it faces certain limitations (PKB interviews, 2024):

- **Limited Data Source:** only from public healthcare providers and General Practitioners (GPs), so excluding other sources, such as private healthcare providers

- **Restricted Data Input**: Patients cannot directly input their own health data, relying entirely on information provided by healthcare professionals
- **Lack of Information Sharing Mechanism**: There is no mechanism for patients to share their health information with caregivers or family members

Published outcomes - statistics

Unfortunately, we couldn't find any statistics about the use of Clicsalud in Andalucia. If you have access to this information or can put us in touch with someone who has, please contact us at book@phr4gov.org.

Screenshots

Screenshots are available on our website, phrs4govs.org.

Bibliography

- Servicio Andaluz de Salud, n.d. What is ClicSalud+. Available at: https://www.sspa.juntadeandalucia.es/servicioanda-luzdesalud/clicsalud/pages/anonimo/ayuda/clicsalud.jsf (accessed: 5 September 2023).

- Servicio Andaluz de Salud, n.d. ClicSalud+. Available at: https://www.sspa.juntadeandalucia.es/servicioanda-luzdesalud/clicsalud/ (accessed: 5 September 2023).

SPAIN – CATALONIA

History

La Meva Salut started in 2009, and all Catalans had access in 2012. Initial use of the platform was low, primarily due to the requirement of a digital certificate, which few people had. Various identity verification alternatives were explored to simplify access while meeting legal and security requirements.

Primary care centres' face-to-face identity verification provided the best solution. A 2014 pilot test provided the username and password system in 33 of the 400 basic health areas (ABS). Access more than tripled, so the rollout was spread to all primary care areas in Catalonia in May 2015 (Aanestad et al., 2017).

Features

La Meva Salut covers care received within Catalonia's health system. The services and information available to patients include:

- Details of their primary care team, including the assigned doctor and nurse, with the option to change doctor.
- Diagnostics and clinical reports covering emergency care, admissions, ambulatory care, test results, and medical notices for work leave and return to work.
- A record of administered vaccines and immunisations.
- The patient's current medication plan.
- A personal agenda showing scheduled tests and visits to primary care centres and hospitals (where this service is integrated).
- Information on the waiting list for any pending surgeries.

- Access to the will document (if the patient has registered one).
- The ability to express the intent to become an organ and tissue donor.
- Use of eConsulta to communicate with healthcare professionals for non-urgent matters that do not require face-to-face contact.
- The ability to schedule appointments, including for international vaccinations.
- The option to securely download clinical information in a coded format using the Health Data to Share feature.

Feature availability depends on the healthcare provider (e.g., hospitals or primary care centres). The patient's provider is determined by their place of residence. Data integration is gradual, relying on healthcare centres within the Comprehensive Health System for Public Use of Catalonia (SISCAT) to continue contributing information (Generalitat de Catalunya, n.d.).

Challenges and areas for improvement

Despite the many benefits of La Meva Salut, there are still some areas where the platform faces challenges and limitations (PKB interviews, 2024):

- **Limited Data Input**: Patients are unable to add personal medical data directly into the system.
- **Exclusively Public Healthcare Data**: La Meva Salut exclusively relies on data provided by Public Healthcare providers.

Published outcomes - statistics

Unfortunately, we couldn't find any statistics about the use of La Meva Salut in Catalonia. If you have access to this information or can put us in touch with someone who has, please contact us at book@phr4gov.org.

Screenshots

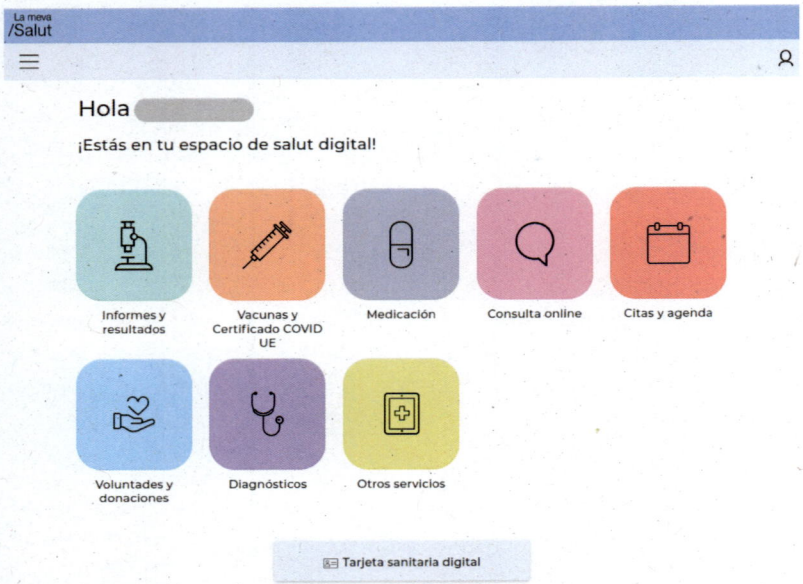

Figure 186. The Home Page provides patients with links to essential areas of the platform. These links include access to test results, vaccination records, COVID certificates, and medication information. Patients can also schedule and attend online consultations, view an appointment calendar, and manage their will and organ donation preferences. Additionally, they can access diagnostic information, explore other services, and view a digital version of their health card.

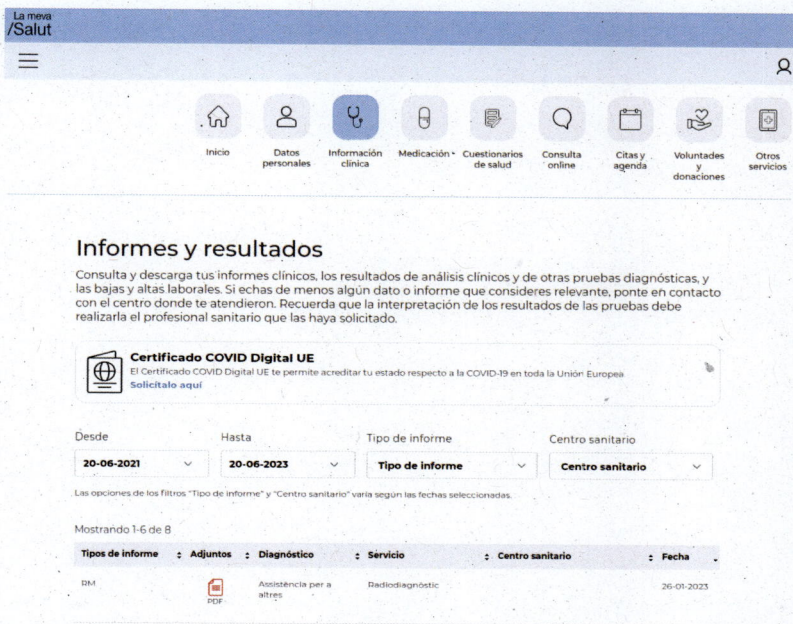

Figure 187. The Information and Results page enables patients to see their clinical test results, imaging findings, and other diagnostic evidence. For each entry, patients can see the type of result, its date, and a PDF to read the full details.

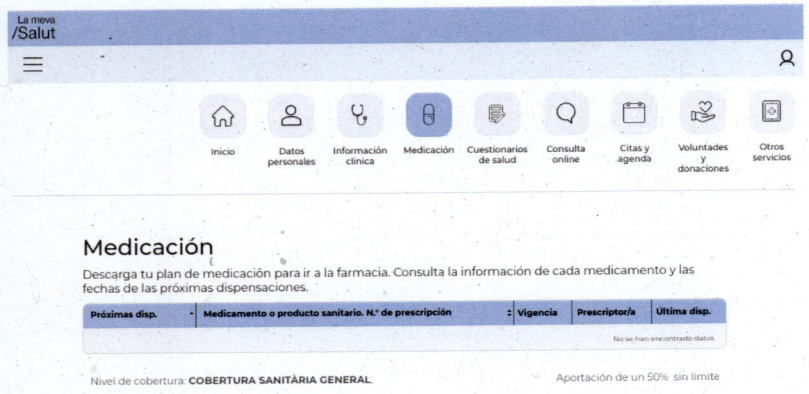

Figure 188. The Medications section allows patients to download their prescription documents, which they can then take to the pharmacy for dispensing. Patients can view key details for each prescription, including the medication name, the prescription duration, the prescriber's name, and the next scheduled refill date.

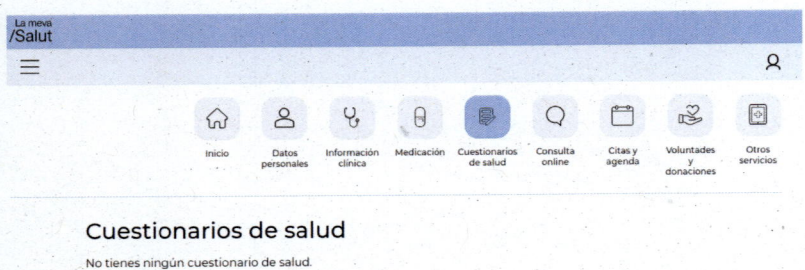

Figure 189. The Health Questionnaires section serves as a tool for gathering information and monitoring health status through patient responses. These questionnaires enable patients to self-assess symptoms, quality of life, and other aspects of their perceived health. Patients can review questionnaires they have previously completed and access any that are awaiting a response.

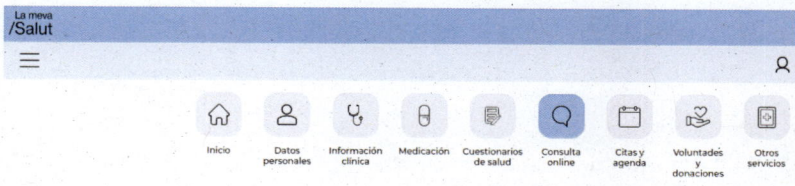

Consulta online

Haz consultas a los profesionales sanitarios, en cualquier momento y sin desplazamientos, a través del servicio de eConsulta. Cuando el profesional haya respondido tu consulta, recibirás una notificación.

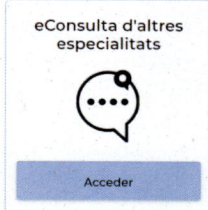

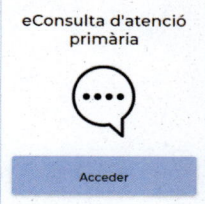

Figure 190. eConsulta enables patients to communicate remotely with profession-als. Patients can submit inquiries, attach files such as documents or images, and receive responses. Professionals can use eConsulta to reply. La Meva Salut sends a notification via email or SMS to the patient about new replies. Not all primary centres currently offer this service. eConsulta of Specialties is available once a special-ised care activates for a patient. The patients can communicate for initial consul-tations and follow-up care after a referral until the patient is discharged. Patients can also request a variety of reports and certificates, including health reports, sick leave reports, medication plan renewals, and more.

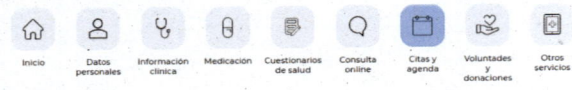

Solicitud de citas y consultas

Haz consultas, gestiones o pide cita con tus profesionales de atención primaria seleccionando el motivo que más se ajusta a tu necesidad.

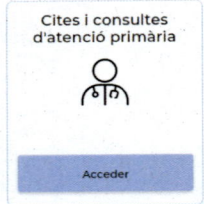

Cites i consultes
d'atenció primària

Acceder

Agenda

Consulta las visitas que tienes programadas. Es posible que no se muestren todas tus visitas. Los centros sanitarios se están incorporando progresivamente a la agenda integrada.

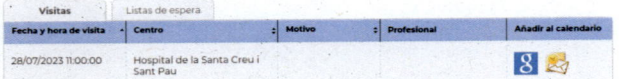

Visitas	Listas de espera			
Fecha y hora de visita	**Centro**	**Motivo**	**Profesional**	**Añadir al calendario**
28/07/2023 11:00:00	Hospital de la Santa Creu i Sant Pau			

Figure 191. Appointments and Agenda allow patients to book appointments by specifying the reason for the visit and the type of professional (e.g., GP or another healthcare professional). Patients can see a list of upcoming appointments and check their status on any waiting lists. Appointment booking is not yet available everywhere as healthcare facilities gradually integrate with the platform.

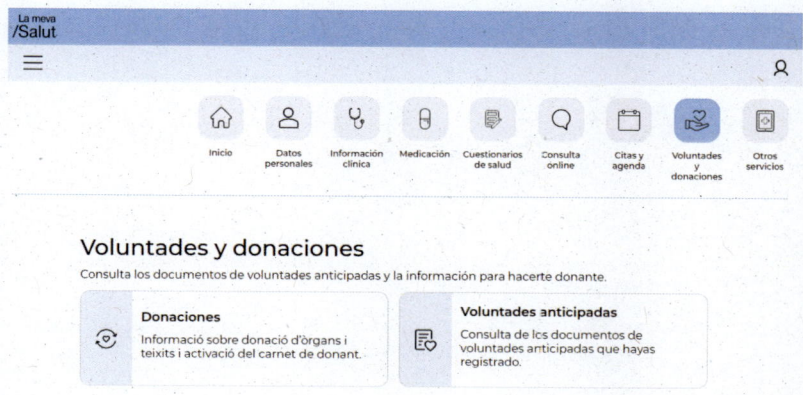

Figure 192. Declaration of Will and Donations allows patients to register their organ donation decisions and to access documents related to their will. Patients can instruct while they have mental capacity what they wish if they lose that capacity. This includes euthanasia and delegating to someone else to make decisions. This legal document is enforceable in all healthcare centres (public and private) as well as in court.

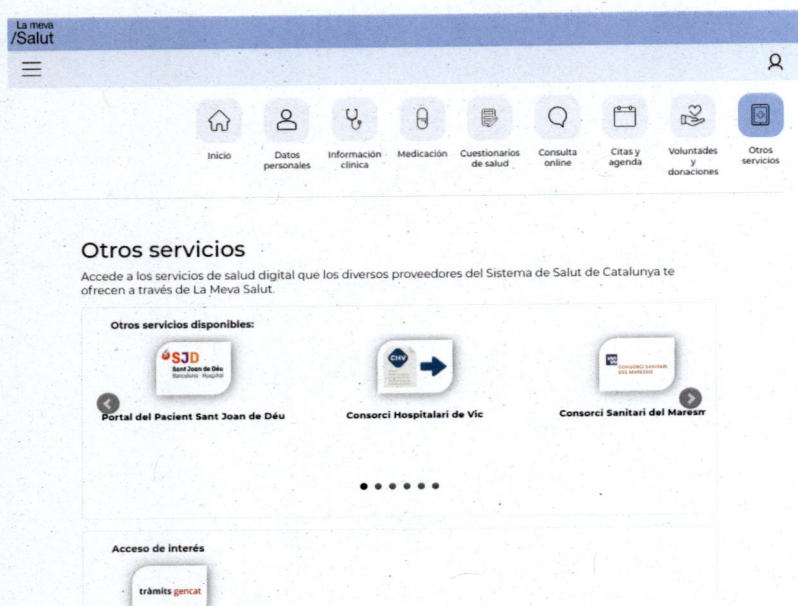

Figure 193. In the Campaigns area, patients can explore promotional initiatives for various products and services. The Other Services section allows patients to explore what health centres offer. Each service opens in a new browser window and operates outside of La Meva Salut.

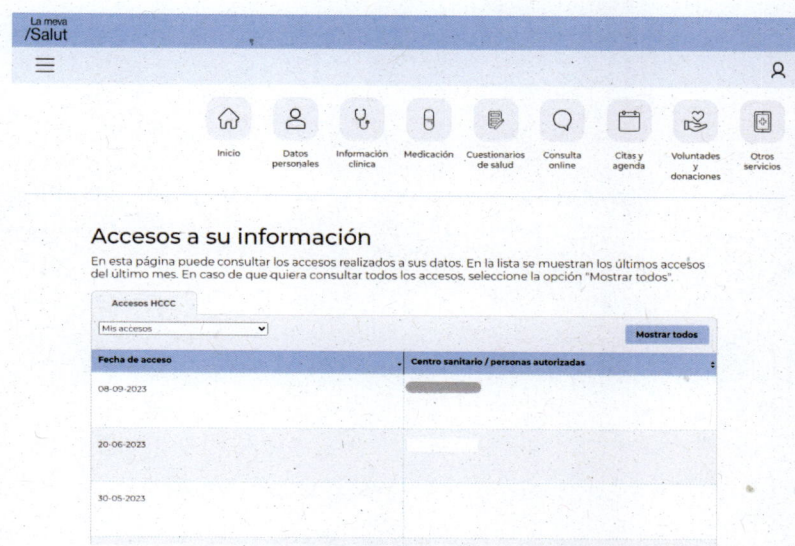

Figure 194. The Access Log Area shows who accessed their health record and when.

Bibliography

- Aanestad, M., Grisot, M., Hanseth, O. and Vassilakopoulou, P., 2017. *Information infrastructures within European health care: Working with the installed base*. Available at: https://library.oapen.org/bitstream/handle/20.500.12657/27913/1002086.pdf (accessed: 8 August 2023).

- Generalitat de Catalunya, n.d. La Meva Salut. Available at: https://catsalut.gencat.cat/ca/serveis-sanitaris/la-meva-salut/index.html#googtrans(ca%7Cen) (accessed: 8 August 2023).

SWEDEN

The rare disease of Mohammad, one of the co-authors of this book, was possible due to its discovery through a Swedish registry. Sweden has pioneered medical registries with long-term health records of all citizens spanning decades. The National Patient Register, for example, has all inpatient stays since 1964. Transparency for the public good is part of Swedish culture; it is why the country was the first to have a Freedom of Information Act back in 1766.

Country's healthcare system in a nutshell

The Swedish healthcare system is decentralised: the 21 regions are responsible for care provision and can decide whether to contract public or private providers. The system is publicly funded and covers all the people who are residents of Sweden, regardless of nationality. 85% of its financing is from regional taxes, complemented by direct federal government transfers.

The system is structured into three administrative tiers (eHealth in Sweden, 2024):

- The **national government** establishes health and medical care principles and guidelines, setting policy priorities through laws, ordinances, or agreements with the Swedish Association of Local Authorities and Regions (SKR).
- The **21 regions** organize health and medical care to ensure universal access.
- The **290 municipalities** handle care for the elderly, individuals with physical and mental disabilities, post-therapy support, and school health care.

Two important pillars of the eHealth strategy in Sweden are E-häl-somyndigheten (eHM), which is the Swedish eHealth Agency, and Inera AB, a company owned by all Regions, Municipalities, and Swedish Association of Local Authorities and Regions (SKR). These two are distinct entities that occasionally collaborate.

- The Swedish eHealth Agency is a government entity dedicated to digitalizing and enhancing the exchange of information among patients, the healthcare system, and pharmacies within the country (Welcome to the Swedish eHealth Agency, 2024). The Agency focuses on e-prescriptions and was also tasked by the Ministry of Social Welfare to create the COVID-19 certification during the pandemic. Its responsibilities are:
    - Carrying out the government's e-health initiatives.
    - Storing digital prescriptions from doctors and forwarding them to pharmacies.
    - Offering Medicine Check service. This allows patients to see information about their prescriptions and whether they are eligible for the high-cost protection card (to avoid paying for medicines for a set period).
    - Collecting information about the quantities of which medicines were sold in Sweden.
    - Offering the Electronic Expert Support service to help pharmacies check whether prescription medicines work together.
- Inera is a "digitization company that, on behalf of municipalities and regions, contributes to the development of welfare." Inera's eHealth strategy is based on (Inera, 2024):
    - National Patient Overview (NPÖ), which allows healthcare providers to see and share patient information securely across different regions.

○   1177 and Journalen, which are designed to offer support and engage citizens.

The remainder of this chapter will focus on 1177, with particular emphasis on Journalen, which serves as Sweden's national Personal Health Record (PHR).

Public vs private

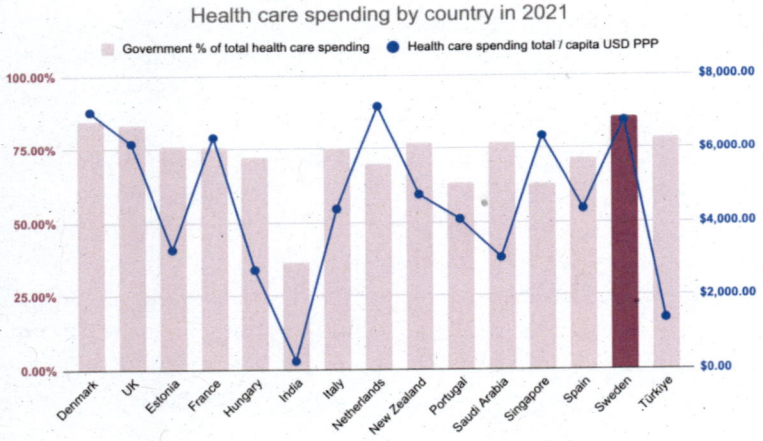

Figure 195. Source: The World Bank. The pink column refers to the public expenditure as a % of the country's total healthcare expenditure. The blue dot is the country's expenditure on health per capita, expressed in international dollars at purchasing power parity.

The national PHR

History

The national patient portal 1177.se is managed by Inera AB (Cijvat, Cornet, and Hägglund, 2021). The portal comprises three key components: a telephone advice service (1177 on the phone), a web-based information platform (1177.se on the web), and a Personal Health Record. The latter, accessible through e-ID authentication, is called Journalen and serves as the national Personal Health Record in Sweden (Hägglund, Blease & Scandurra, 2020).

Journalen integrates Electronic Health Record (EHR) information from various systems used by Swedish healthcare organisations through a national health information exchange platform. Initially launched as a project in the Uppsala region, its success inspired other regions, and they asked to adopt it. As a result of this, Uppsala transferred the project to Inera for national management. The first region connected to this infrastructure in 2012, with the final joining in 2018. Despite this widespread adoption, features still vary depending on the region and the healthcare provider (Hägglund, Scandurra 2022). Today, Journalen serves as a centralised access point, connecting EHR systems across all 21 regions in Sweden.

eHealth is deeply embedded in Sweden's healthcare system, with annual investments of around $1.22 billion in healthcare IT across all regions. Electronic health record solutions are universally adopted, with 99% of prescriptions issued electronically. The COVID-19 pandemic further accelerated the adoption of digital health services, with digital consultations doubling in 2020, representing 11% of all medical appointments.

In collaboration with the Swedish Association of Local Authorities and Regions (SKR), the Swedish government has outlined a vision for its national eHealth strategy. By 2025, the country aims at becoming a global leader in utilising digitalisation and eHealth to enhance health and welfare while promoting individuals' independence (International Trade Administration, U.S. Department of Commerce, 2023).

Sweden's healthcare data exchange, National Service Platform (NTjP), receives data source systems. These include local EHRs and larger regional databases. Information such as lab results, vaccinations, and diagnoses flows into the NTjP via APIs from regional databases and other authorised systems.

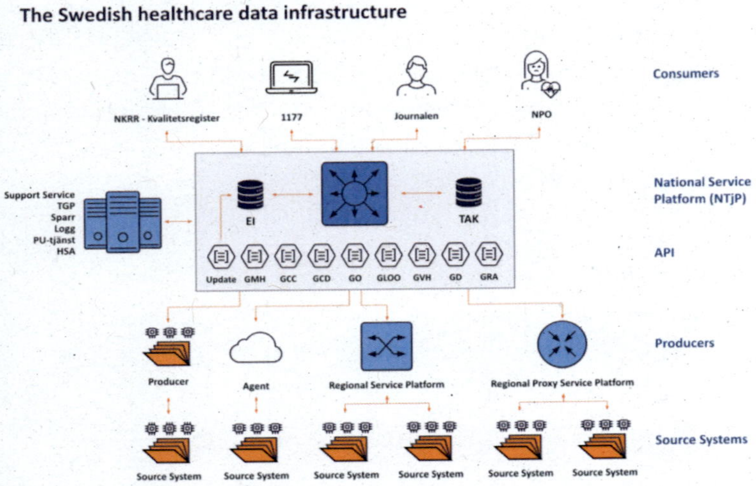

The Swedish healthcare data infrastructure

Figure 196. National Service Platform (NTjP) is the centre of Sweden's healthcare data infrastructure (PKB interviews, 2024)

An electronic directory that contains data about healthcare organisations and personnel, such as clinicians, operating across the country. This is on the left in a blue box.

Consumer platforms like 1177 and Journalen provide patients with access to their health information. They are at the top of the diagram.

Private healthcare providers are source systems on the bottom left. They cannot directly connect to the NTjP because they are private. Their tech company (or a third-party company) can apply to become an agent for Inera.

Agents connect systems to Inera's infrastructure and ensure the technical requirements are met for healthcare providers to use Inera's services. Agents themselves do not use the services but enable healthcare providers to send data to platforms like Journalen. Notably, private providers can only send data for services funded by tax money. So, self-funded procedures (e.g., cosmetic surgery) are excluded.

Being an agent typically costs more than regional access, but many regions require this connection when contracting private providers. Additionally, agents have limited access to certain services.

Features

The bibliography for this section is from 2018, and we were unable to locate more recent information.

Within the Journalen system, patients can access the following (Moll et al., 2018):

- Medical notes from the EHRs from all healthcare professionals and connected healthcare providers (both public and private) who have agreed to give access.
- A list of prescribed medications.
- Laboratory results.
- Warnings.
- Diagnoses.
- Maternity care records.
- Referrals.
- Vaccination records.

In some regions, users can also access a log function, allowing them to see who has viewed their record.

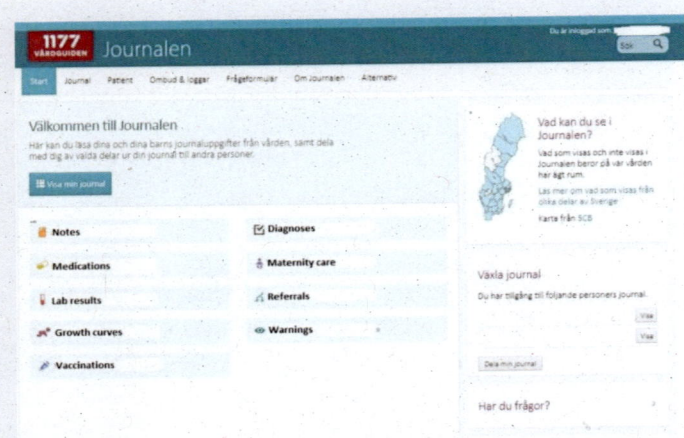

Figure 1. The patient-accessible electronic health record Journalen after log-in, showing the functions and information available (partially translated). Licensed under fair use. Source: https://e-tjanster.1177.se/. Service produced by Inera AB under the auspices of Swedish county councils and regions.

Figure 197. Source: Moll et al., 2018.

	Medical Notes	Diag-noses	Visits (time/date / provider)	Lab Results	Medi-cations	Immuni-zations	Referrals	Medical alerts	Access Log Lists	Psychi-atry	Health Declaration Forms	Blocking of record	TOTAL
Blekinge													6
Dalarna													3
Gotland													0
Gävleborg													0
Halland													5
Jämtland/Härjedalen													0
Jönköping													3
Kalmar													4
Kronoberg													3
Norrbotten													4
Skåne													4
Stockholm													4
Södermanland													4
Uppsala													9
Värmland													6
Västerbotten													4
Västernorrland													0
Västmanland													3
VGR													4
Örebro													6
Östergötland													7
Capio (private care provider)													4
TOTAL of regions (of 20)	18	15	12	8	7	7	5	4	3	2	1	1	

Figure 2. Information shown in Journalen depending on county council or health care provider (blue squares) during the time of the survey.

Figure 198. Source: Moll et al., 2018.

234

Challenges and areas for improvement

Data fragmentation is a significant challenge for Journalen, as various EHR systems are in use across the country. Despite the national Health Information Exchange platform efforts, challenges remain in achieving a comprehensive overview of health data. Variability in information accessibility among care providers—due to differing policies and regulations—results in a fragmented patient view, depending on the location, timing, and purpose of seeking treatment. This issue is closely tied to the difficulty in agreeing on a national regulatory framework for patients' direct access to their health information.

Resistance to change among healthcare professionals also poses challenges. Many professionals are concerned about how the system might impact their work. Key worries include an increase in workload, as more time may be required to explain EHR contents and address patient queries. Some professionals also fear that patient access to EHRs could lead to misunderstandings, misinterpretations, and conflicts, potentially causing unnecessary anxiety for patients (Hägglund, 2017).

A 2022 survey on the usability of the Swedish Personal Health Record highlighted several additional concerns (Hägglund and Scandurra, 2022):

- Different regions offer distinct features and provide varying levels of health information to patients.
- Some regions did not provide access to past health information, only to data from the date the region launched the portal.
- Many regions impose restrictions on patient access to specific clinical data, such as mental health records. Some respondents felt discriminated against due to the limited access to their mental health information.

- When a child turns 13, parents lose access to the child's record, yet the child cannot access their own record until they turn 16. This results in a three-year period where neither the parent nor the child can see the record.
- The platform lacks a messaging feature, preventing patients and healthcare professionals from communicating with each other remotely.

The following table, from Cijvat, Cornet, and Hägglund, 2021 (Table 4), shows "Barriers on the local implementation level":

Category	Sweden	Netherlands
Systems and suppliers	Technical limitations of systems. High costs for connecting small EHR systems. Testing prior to implementation is necessary. Difficult requisites for connecting to the HIE.	Limitations in choice and possibilities of systems. Large dependency on software suppliers. Alignment of systems necessary but difficult. Systems and suppliers determine the achievement of VIPP (the VIPP programme is an initiative in the Netherlands designed to enhance the exchange of information between patients and healthcare professionals).

Social and organisational	Resistance and fears from physicians. Changing healthcare providers' routines, workflows, and attitudes.	Physicians' reluctance, resistance, and fears. Changing healthcare providers' political status and workflow. Effects on hospitals' culture and work processes. Concerns for patients' confusion, questions, and fears. Gradual implementation is necessary to keep physicians on board.
Resources	High costs for connecting to HIE. Time-consuming decision-making due to flexibility in the national regulatory framework.	VIPP requires a lot of human work. Human work leads to high costs. Too little time to make VIPP's deadlines.
Policies, laws, and regulations		Some VIPP goals are challenging to accomplish.

		Strict privacy regulations are not in patients' interests. Strict security rules impede user-friendliness.
Governance	A gradual approach is necessary to get all stakeholders on board. Flexibility in choosing EHR systems in some countries, but only one supported.	Gradual implementation to keep physicians on board. VIPP has no or low priority.

The following table from Cijvat, Cornet, and Hägglund, 2021 (Table 3) shows *"Barriers on the national level"*:

Category	Sweden	Netherlands
Systems and suppliers	Authentication methods.	Difficulties in measuring hospitals' progress.
Social and organisational	Resistance and fears from physicians.	-
Resources	Financing the development of Journalen. Too little time to take precautions for physicians' resistance.	-

Policies, laws, and regulations	Include electable rules to make progress. Electable rules caused confusion and inequality for users. Giving patients direct online access to records was illegal when Journalen was first introduced in 2002.	Challenging to define goals adequately for desired outcomes. Challenging to estimate reasonable usage percentages. Slow development of other national programs.
Effect of barriers	Delays. Restrictions on information that is displayed.	Delays.

Published outcomes - statistics

Unfortunately, we couldn't find any statistics about the use of the Swedish PHR. If you have access to this information or can put us in touch with someone who has, please contact us at book@phr4gov.org.

Screenshots

Unfortunately, we couldn't find any screenshots of the Swedish PHR. If you have access to this information or can put us in touch with someone who has, please contact us at book@phr4gov.org.

Bibliography

- Cijvat, C.D., Cornet, R. and Hägglund, M., 2021. Factors influencing development and implementation of patients' access to electronic health records—a comparative study of Sweden and the Netherlands. Frontiers in Public Health, 9, p.621210. (online). Available at: https://www.frontiersin.org/journals/public-health/articles/10.3389/fpubh.2021.621210/full (accessed: 3 May 2023).

- eHealth in Sweden, n.d. GNIUS. Edited by Délégation au numérique en santé (Ministerial delegation for Digital Health). Available at: https://gnius.esante.gouv.fr/en/international-digital-health-systems/ehealth-in-sweden (accessed: 3 May 2023).

- Hägglund, M., 2017. Electronic health records in Sweden—how can we go from transparency to collaboration? Thebmjopinion. (online) 23 June. Available at: https://blogs.bmj.com/bmj/2017/06/23/maria-hagglund-electronic-health-records-in-sweden-how-can-we-go-transparency-to-collaboration/ (accessed: 2 August 2024).

- Hägglund, M., 2020. Mobile access and adoption of the Swedish National Patient Portal. In: A. Värri et al., eds. Integrated Citizen Centered Digital Health and Social Care. The European Federation for Medical Informatics (EFMI) and IOS Press. Available at: https://www.diva-portal.org/smash/get/diva2:1509909/FULLTEXT01.pdf (accessed: 3 May 2023).

- Hägglund, M. and Scandurra, I., 2022. Usability of the Swedish accessible electronic health record: qualitative survey study. JMIR Human Factors, 9(2), p.e37192. (online) Available at: https://humanfactors.jmir.org/2022/2/e37192 (accessed: 3 May 2023).

- Inera, 2024. Inera. Available at: https://www.inera.se/ (accessed: 14 November 2024).

- International Trade Administration, U.S. Department of Commerce, 2023. Sweden - Country Commercial Guide. (online)

Available at: https://www.trade.gov/country-commercial-guides/sweden-ehealth (accessed: 3 May 2023).

- Moll, J., Rexhepi, H., Cajander, Å., Grünloh, C., Huvila, I., Hägglund, M., Myreteg, G., Scandurra, I. and Åhlfeldt, R.M., 2018. Patients' experiences of accessing their electronic health records: national patient survey in Sweden. Journal of Medical Internet Research, 20(11), p.e278. (online) Available at: https://www.jmir.org/2018/11/e278/ (accessed: 3 May 2023).

- Welcome to the Swedish eHealth Agency, n.d. eHälsomyndigheten. Available at: https://www.ehalsomyndigheten.se/languages/english/welcome-to-the-swedish-ehealth-agency/ (accessed: 3 May 2023).

TÜRKIYE

Turkish Airlines flies to the largest number of countries (Wikipedia, 2025). "Turkish hairlines" is the name of the hair transplant industry of Türkiye. A million people came in 2022 and spent approximately $2 billion (TRT World, 2023). This is part of the country's growth and internationalisation, which is powered by a dynamic private sector.

Country's healthcare system in a nutshell

Türkiye provides universal public health insurance through the Social Security Institution (SSI), allowing all registered residents access to free healthcare.

However, equitable access remains a challenge, partly due to a nationwide shortage of doctors. As a result, many people opt for additional private insurance to cover treatments in private hospitals.

The Republic of Türkiye Ministry of Health is responsible for setting health policy and owns more than half of the country's hospitals. The SSI handles collecting and pooling social security premiums, contracts with healthcare providers and sets tariffs for services. Other government agencies manage workforce planning and the regulation of drugs and medical devices.

Funding for social insurance premiums comes from both employer and employee contributions, with exemptions for those on low incomes. The Ministry of Health contracts with family physicians for preventative and primary care, paying according to the number of patients under care. Patients are required to make co-payments at varying levels for primary, secondary, and tertiary care services (World Health Organization, 2024).

According to the most recent data from 2011, health insurance covered 86% of the population in Türkiye. This coverage encompasses both those who are members of health insurance schemes and those who have free access to state-provided healthcare services (Our World in Data, n.p.).

Public vs private

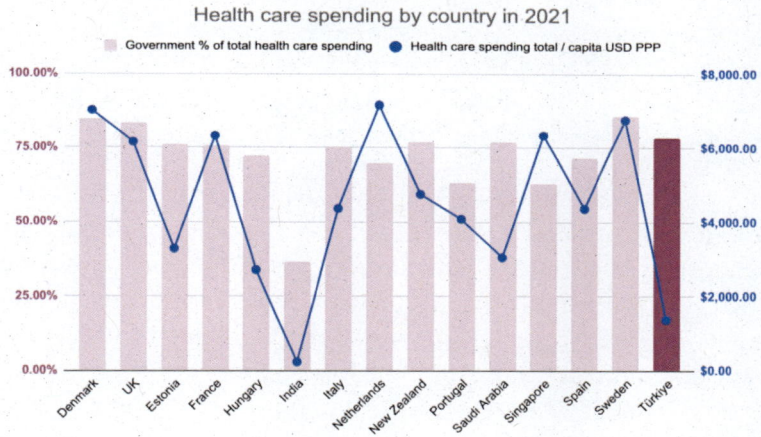

Figure 199. Source: The World Bank. The pink column refers to the public expenditure as a % of the country's total healthcare expenditure. The blue dot is the country's expenditure on health per capita, expressed in international dollars at purchasing power parity.

The national PHR

History

In 2008, the Republic of Türkiye Ministry of Health began to centralise and process personal health records, along with administrative and financial data, from all healthcare providers.

This started with the National Health Data Dictionary (NHDD), which has since served as a reference for information systems used by all healthcare facilities, significantly contributing to terminology standardisation. Subsequent steps toward digitalisation were built upon this common terminology and system architecture outlined in the NHDD. The NHDD laid the foundations for the Sağlık ("health") system, introduced in 2009, upgraded to version 2 in 2011, and most recently, the e-Nabız system.

e-Nabız ("e-pulse"), the Türk Personal Health Record, launched in 2015. e-Nabız was developed to enable citizens to access their health data collected from multiple healthcare institutions in one place. Through the platform, patients can also authorise their healthcare professionals to access their records.

The Ministry of Health developed e-Nabiz and used private contractors for professional services for maintenance and technical support of the system (PKB interviews, 2024). Tiga Healthcare Technologies is one of the Ministry's main contractors for this project (Tiga Healthcare Technologies, 2023). The health tech company also holds contracts with the Ministry for the Pharmaceutical Track & Trace System and E-prescription (as shown in the image below).

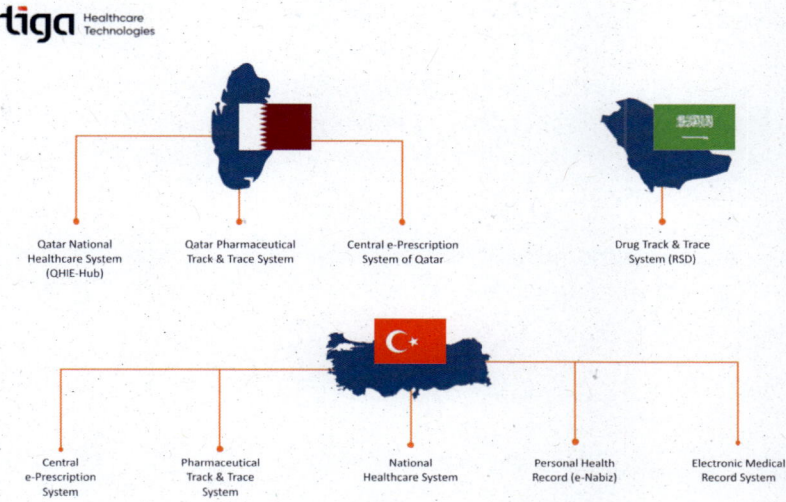

Figure 200

Tiga Health Timeline

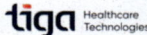

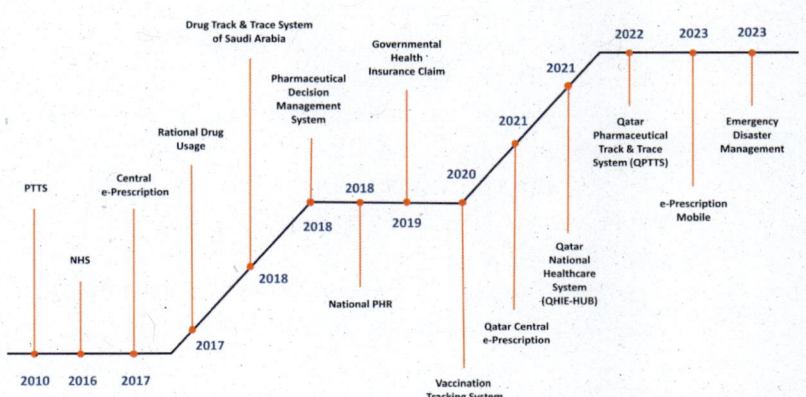

Figure 201

Features

The Türk PHR system, e-Nabiz, has 38 features for treatment, prevention, health promotion, and health-related and interrelated areas. Data sources include both public and private healthcare providers.

- The **appointment** section shows future scheduled hospital appointments and information on past ones. The patient can book new ones. Past visit details include:
    - prescriptions
    - diagnosis
    - written reports
    - tests performed
    - radiological images.
- The notifications section shows recent activities, such as the latest login and hospital visits.
- Patients have multiple options when it comes to sharing:
    - "No physician can see my information"
    - "Family physicians can see my information"
    - "The physician who performed the examination can see my information"
    - " Every physician in the health facility where I had my examination can see my health information"
    - "All physicians can see my information."
- Patients can also share a piece of selected health information with persons of their choice for a period of their choice (they can also share permanently) after entering their email address and phone number to confirm.

Patients can also see:

- Disease history and personal information such as blood type, age, and smoking status
- Measurements such as weight, height, and body mass index
- Allergies

- Intensive care hospitalisation information
- Vaccine calendar
- Access log to check who has accessed their record
- COVID-19 vaccine information and appointments, get the vaccine certification

They can also:

- Evaluate a health facility visit in terms of service quality and comment on the visit
- Track and manage their blood and bone marrow donation choices
- Make organ donation choices
- Let their insurance companies access the data
- Add 'emergency notes' to a section so that healthcare professionals can read them in case of emergency
- Upload files
- Add measurements

e-Nabiz also retrieves data from iOS HealthKit or Google Fit if the patient gives access from their smartphone (Birinci, 2023).

Challenges and areas for improvement

The system lacks a symptom-tracking feature.

Published outcomes - statistics

The research paper titled 'A Digital Opportunity for Patients to Manage Their Health: Türkiye National Personal Health Record System (The e-Nabız)' (Birinci, 2023) provides statistics about its usage and impact:

- **Rapid User Growth**: In 2018, e-Nabız had 11 million users. By 2022, this number had grown to 68 million active users, representing 80% of Türkiye's population.
- **Integrations**: The platform collects data from 28,608 system-integrated health facilities and 39 other public institutions, including ministries.
- **Cost Savings**: Since its launch in 2015, e-Nabız has stored radiological images within the system, eliminating the need for patients to request duplicate copies. This innovation has resulted in a 27.5% reduction in costs, saving 750 million Türk Lira (approximately USD 21.87 million) in radiological imaging expenses from the platform's inception until 2023.

Table 5 from the paper presents e-Nabız usage rates among Türk citizens in 2021, as shown below:

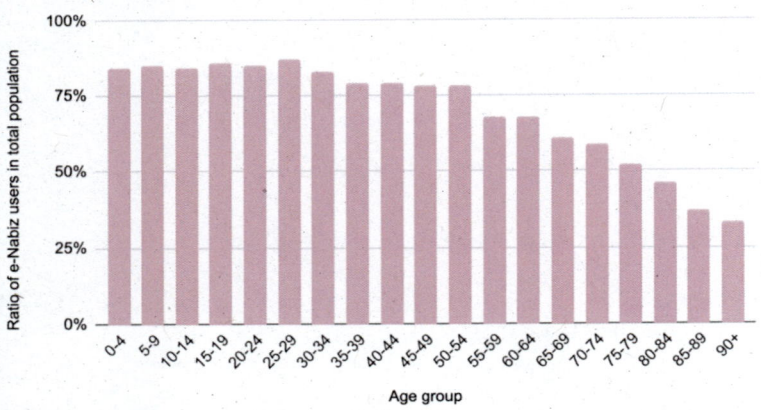

Ratio of e-Nabiz users in total population vs Age group

Figure 202. Usage for children under 15 years old is measured by parental usage (Birinci, 2023)

Screenshots

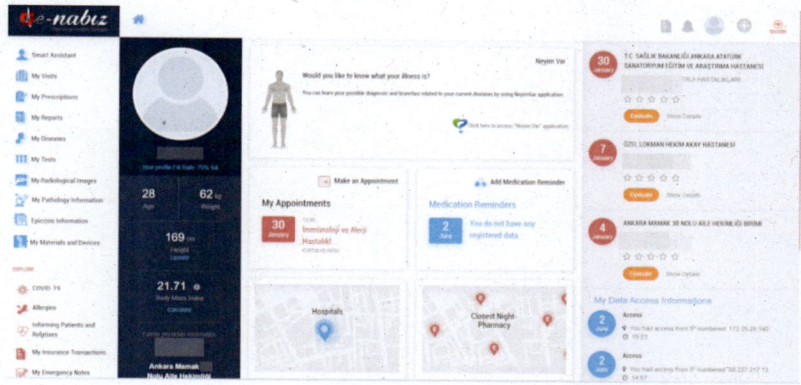

Figure 203. My Medical History Screen (home page).

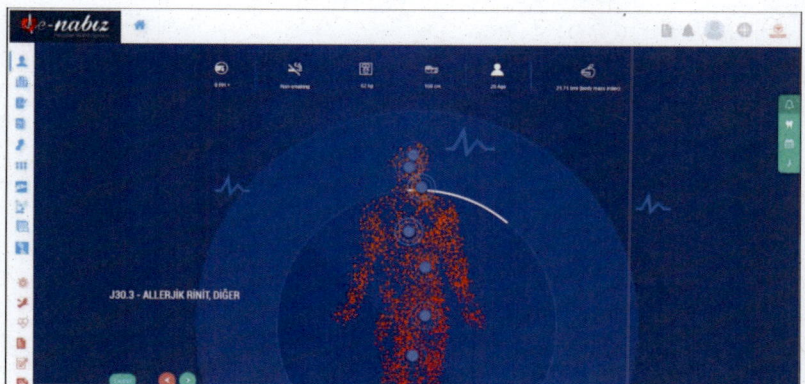

Figure 204. The Smart Assistant Screen can be accessed from the homepage menu. On this page, patients can view their disease history and personal information such as blood type, weight, height, age, body mass index, and smoking status. The diseases they have had are marked on a human body diagram, and the diagnoses are shown in the fields indicated by dots.

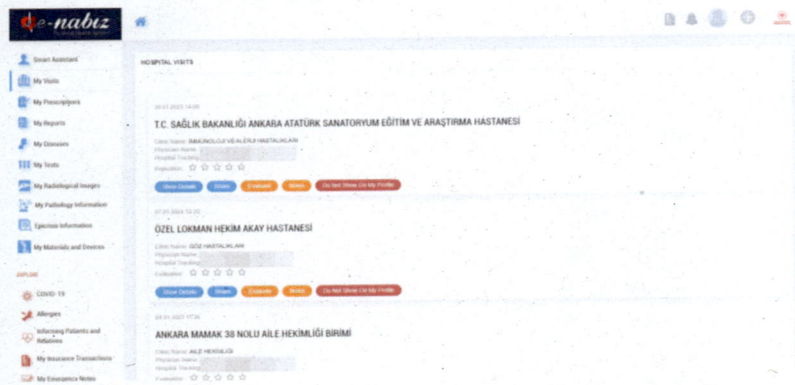

Figure 205. My Health Facility Visits Screen: for each visit, patients can see details and contents of the prescription, diagnosis, report, tests performed, and radiological images taken.

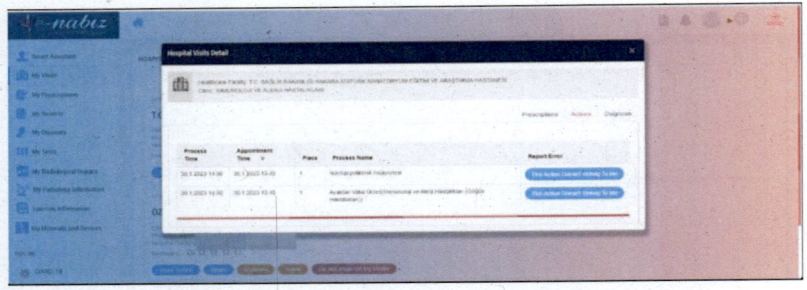

Figure 206. My Visits / Hospital Visits Details Screen.

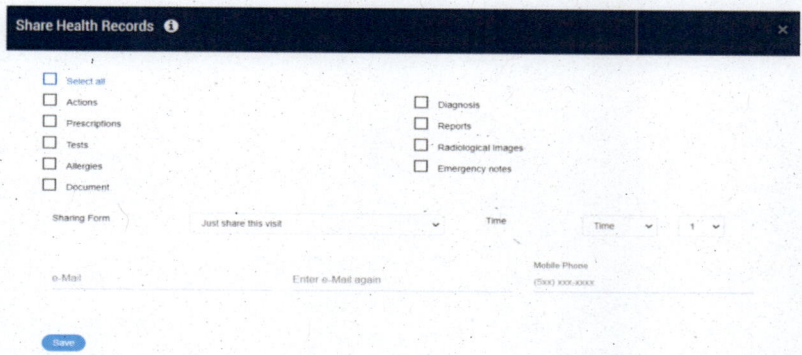

Figure 207. My Visits / Share Health Records Screen: patients can share selected health information for a temporary period to be set by them. They will be sent a verification code.

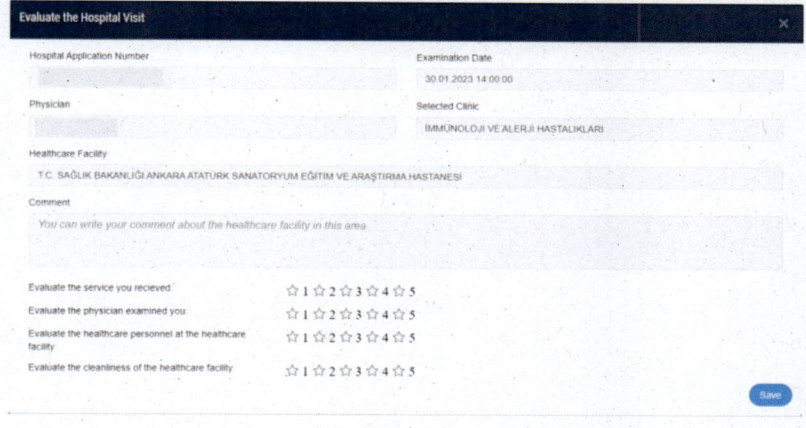

Figure 208. My Visits / Hospital Visit Evaluation Screen: patients can evaluate the health facility in terms of service quality.

251

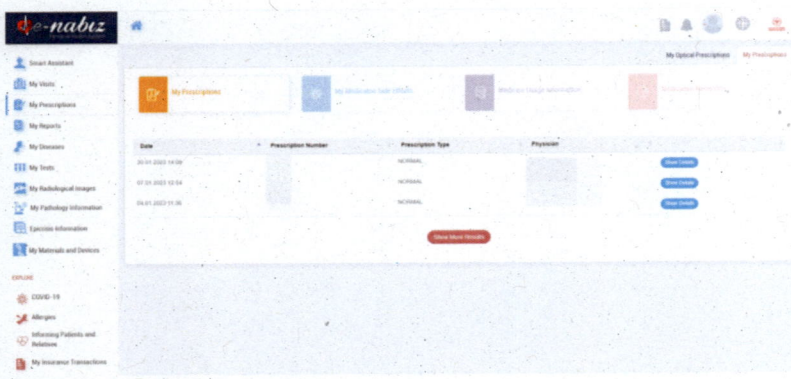

Figure 209. My Prescriptions Screen.

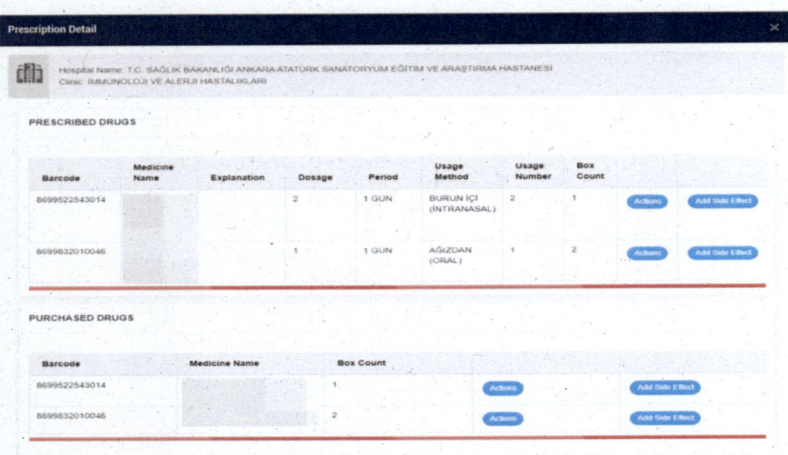

Figure 210. My Prescriptions / Prescription Details Screen.

252

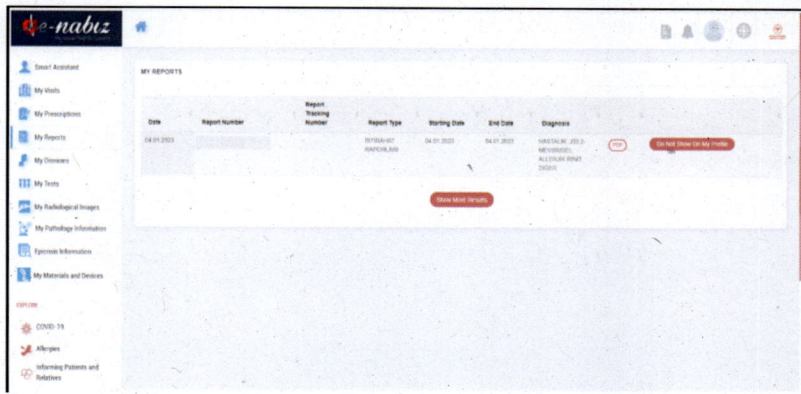

Figure 211. My Reports Screen: here, patients can see all the reports written by their physicians.

O

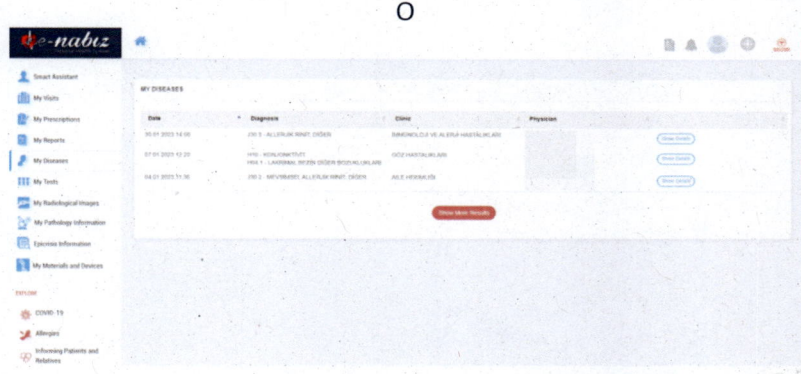

Figure 212. My Diseases Screen (diagnoses).

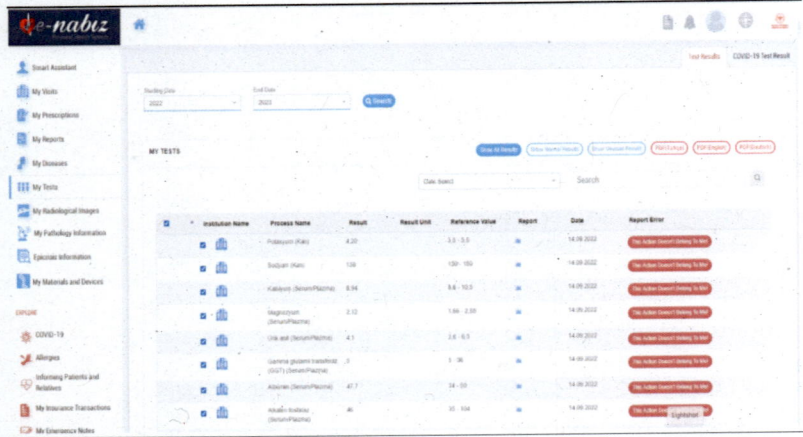

Figure 213. My Tests Screen: patients can see all tests they have had, their results, and their reference values by the date and description, and they can access the details by clicking on the test. They can filter by date range and procedure name.

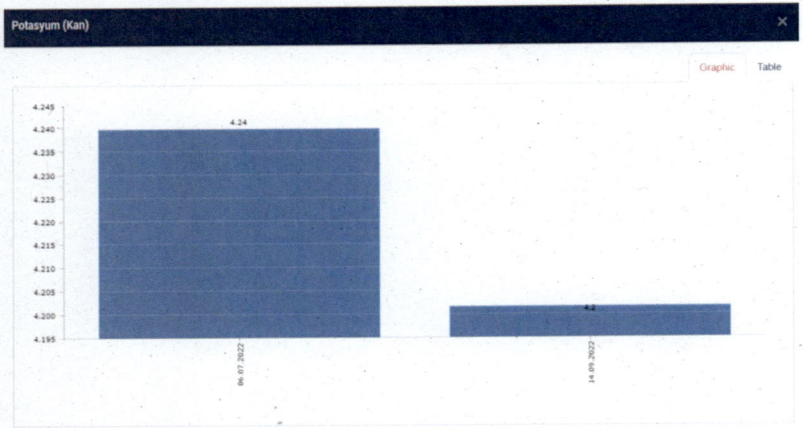

Figure 214. My Tests / Test Results Chart Display Screen.

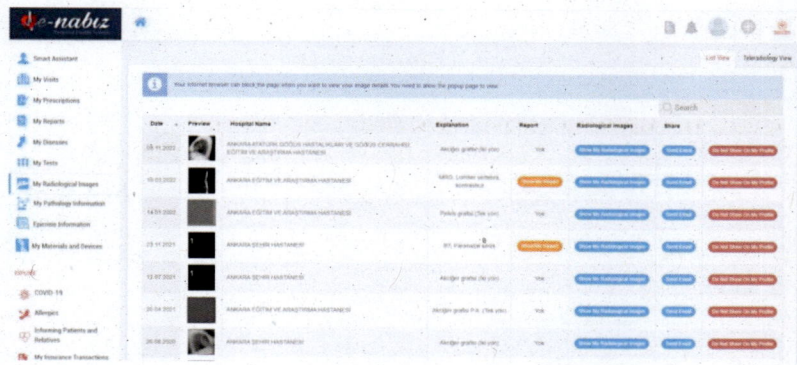

Figure 215. My Radiology Images Screen.

On the **Pathology Information** page, patients can download the report of the pathology procedure that they have undergone in health institutions for the diagnosis of all diseases, treatment options, and determination of diseases associated with genetic syndromes.

On the **'My Epicrisis Information'** page, patients can download epicrisis reports containing information about each of their conditions, their respective diagnoses, and treatments.

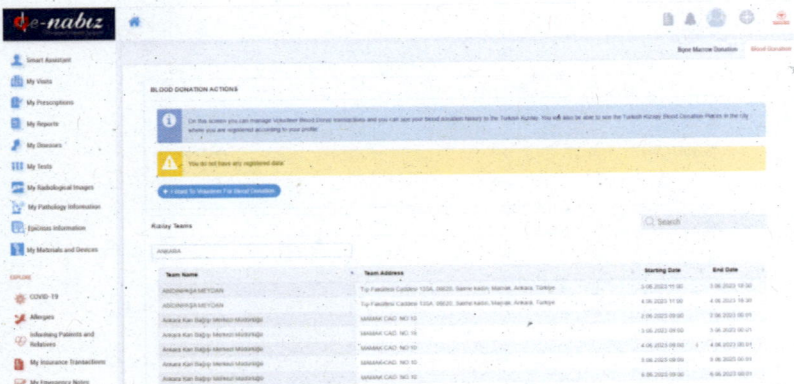

Figure 216. My Blood Donation Screen: patients can view the address and date information of blood donation teams and track their blood donation history.

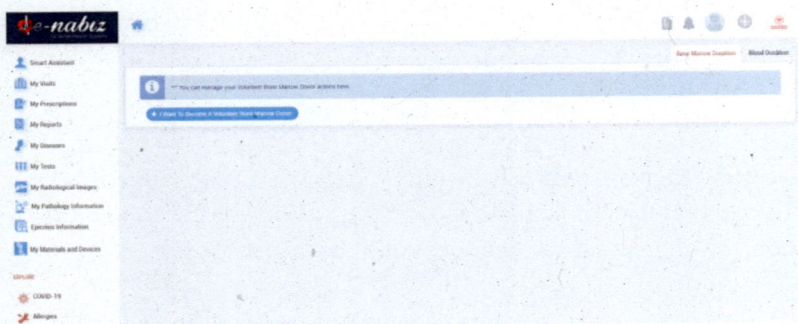

Figure 217. Voluntary Bone Marrow Donation Screen: here, patients can submit their request to become a voluntary bone marrow donor.

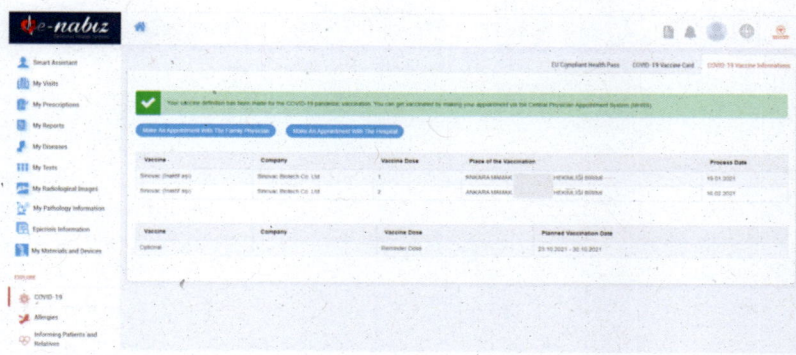

Figure 218. Covid-19 Vaccine Information Screen.

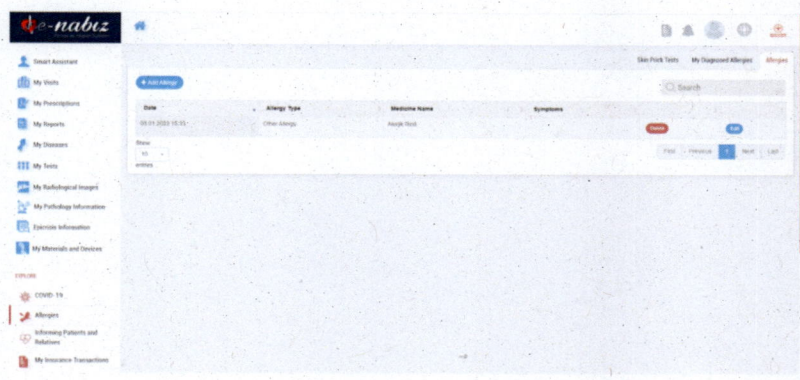

Figure 219. My Allergies Screen: patients can view and add new ones. However, patients cannot add Diagnosed allergies and Skin Prick tests.

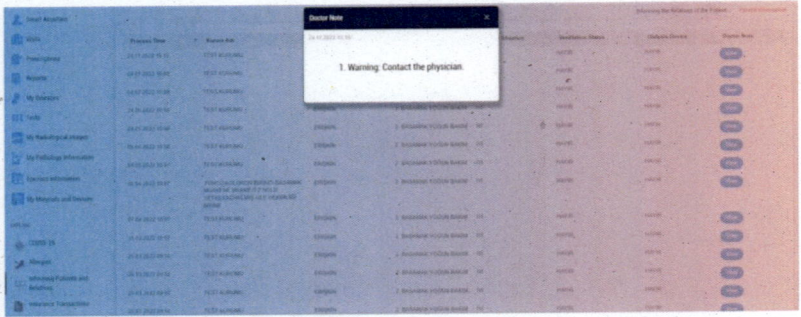

Figure 220. Patient Information Screen. Patients can access the latest status information regarding intensive care hospitalization information about themselves and their consenting relatives, as well as view the physician notes.

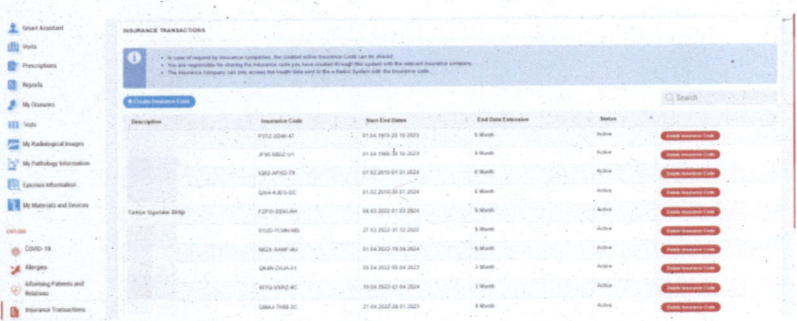

Figure 221. My Insurance Activities Screen: patients can generate an insurance code to allow insurance companies access to their health records. Insurance companies can only view health data submitted to the e-Nabız System using this code. On the "My Insurance Activities" page, patients can enter details of the insurance companies with which the code will be shared. A separate insurance code can be created for each insurance provider, or a single code can be shared with multiple companies.

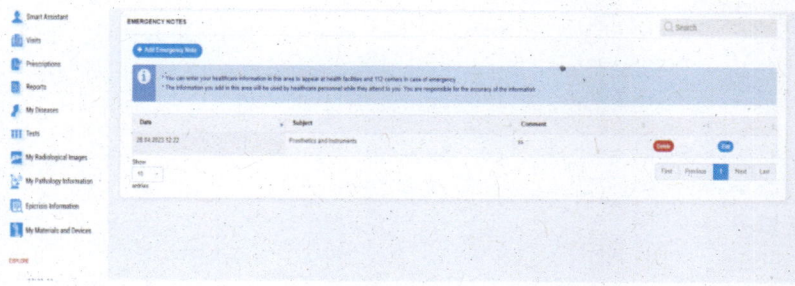

Figure 222. My Emergency Notes Screen: patients can add to this page so that notes are available for healthcare professionals in case of emergency.

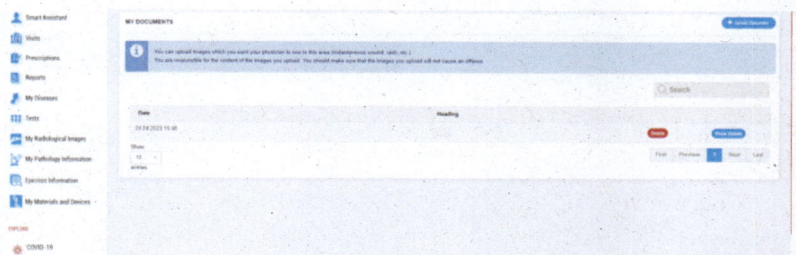

Figure 223. On the 'My Documents' page, patients can upload photos related to their health that they want their physician to see, such as rashes, etc. Once uploaded, the patient is also free to edit or delete the documents.

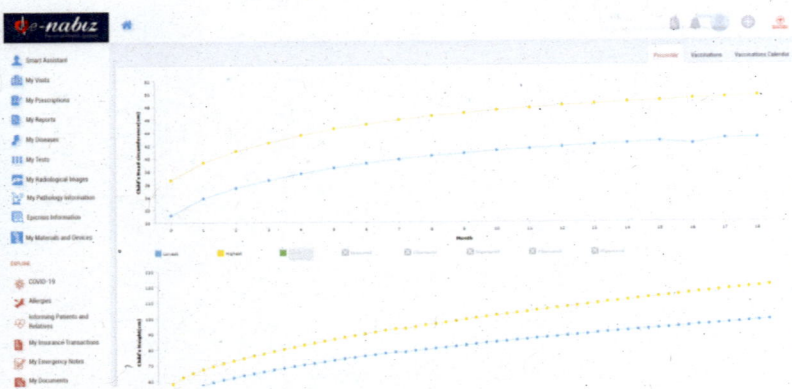

Figure 224. Vaccine Calendar: patients can view their childhood vaccines through the Vaccine Calendar. This feature shows the vaccines included in the childhood immunisation schedule of the Ministry of Health of the Republic of Türkiye, along with their current status. For those needing a document, the Electronic Vaccine Card can be downloaded as a PDF. The Vaccines section also provides a detailed list of all administered vaccines. Patients can access percentile charts for head circumference, height, and weight in the Percentile section.

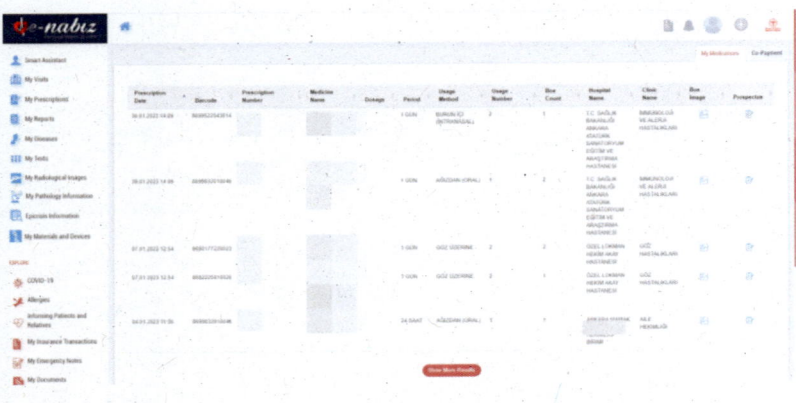

Figure 225. My Medications Screen: patients can see the list of all medications prescribed and details such as dose, period, number of boxes, box picture, package insert, amount of medication contribution due, medication contribution due difference by the substitute medication, amount of examination, and prescription contribution dues.

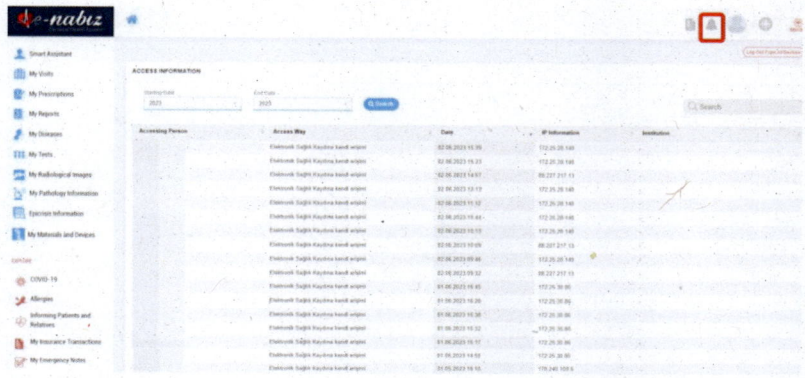

Figure 226. Access log details screen: patients can see who accessed their record, when, and from which institution.

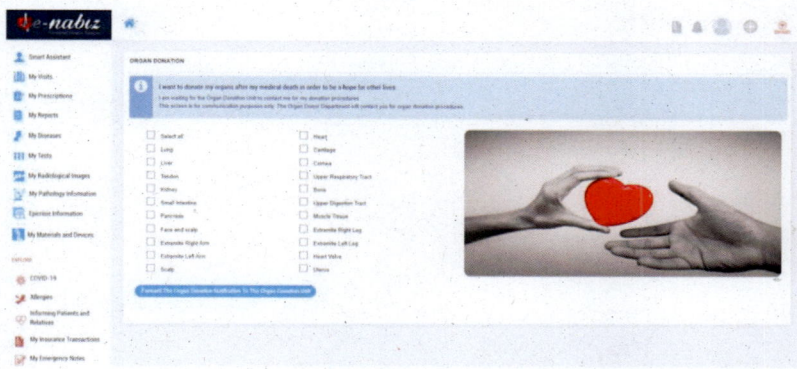

Figure 227. Organ donation choices screen: patients can choose to donate their organs after their death. On this page, they can select which organs to donate.

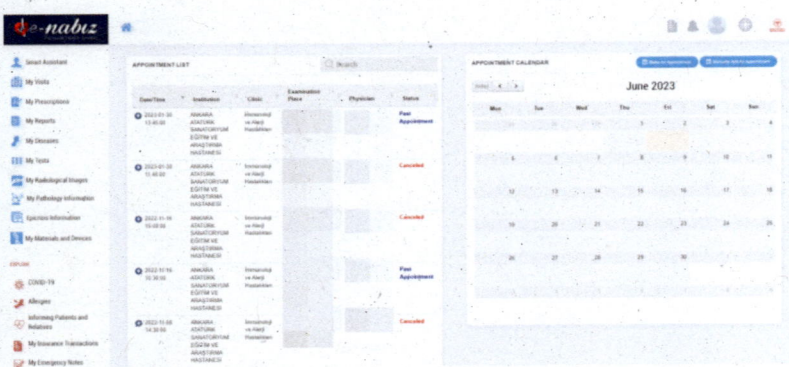

Figure 228. Appointment Activities Screen: patients can book new ones and see those that are already scheduled.

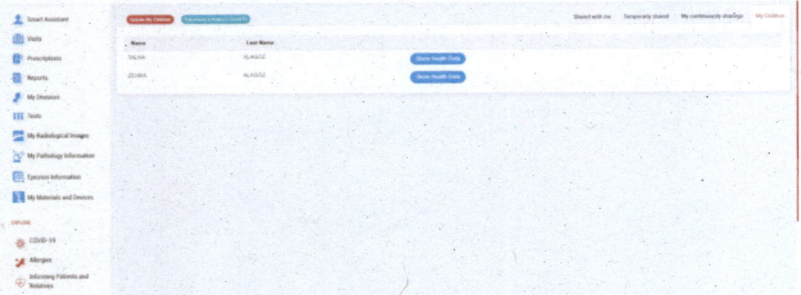

Figure 229. Sharing / My Children Screen: patients can share any part or the entire record. If they have children under 18, they can view their health records in the "My Children" section with the consent of the other parent. In the "Permanently Shared by Me" tab, patients can give any person with permanent access to view their records. Patients can also send messages from the My Messages section. Patients can manage their time-limited permissions with the "Temporarily Shared by Me" tab. From the "Shared with Me" tab, they can access those who have shared their health details with them. They can edit the content of the health details they have shared and revoke the permission. They can accept/reject connection requests.

Bibliography

- Birinci, Ş., 2023. A digital opportunity for patients to manage their health: Turkey national personal health record system (The e-Nabız). Balkan Medical Journal, 40(3), p.215. Available at: https://pmc.ncbi.nlm.nih.gov/articles/PMC10175887/ (accessed: 13 December 2023).

- e-Nabız Has More Than 74 Million Users, 2023(online) Available at: https://www.tigahealth.com/e-nabiz-has-more-than-76-million-us-ers/#:~:text=e%2DNab%C4%B1z%2C%20which%20was%20put,more%20than%2071%20million%20users (accessed: 13 December 2023).

- User Manual e-Nabız, 2024. (pdf) Available at: https://ena-biz.gov.tr/document/User_ManualEN.pdf (accessed: 2 August 2024).

- TRT World, 2023. Hair transplant industry gives Türkiye's medical tourism a $2B boost. TRT World. Available at: https://www.trtworld.com/business/hair-transplant-industry-gives-t%C3%BCrkiye-s-medical-tourism-a-2b-boost-64399(accessed: 21 January 2025).

- Wikipedia, 2025. List of airlines by countries served. Available at: https://en.wikipedia.org/wiki/List_of_airlines_by_countries_served (accessed: 22 January 2025).

- World Health Organization, 2024. Türkiye: Country overview. Available at: https://eurohealthobservatory.who.int/countries/turkiye (accessed: 2 August 2024).

WALES

Evidence-based medicine's founder, Archie Cochrane, started with the health of Welsh coal miners. Working with Welsh miners deepened his commitment to the use of randomized controlled trials to evaluate medical interventions. He observed firsthand the limitations of unproven treatments offered to miners (Cochrane, 1972).

> *After considerable thought, I wrote out my slogan: "All effective treatment must be free."*

Country's healthcare system in a nutshell

Residents of Wales, like all UK residents, have access to public healthcare funded through taxation. Responsibility for healthcare is transferred from the UK central government to each of the devolved nations. The Welsh Government manages the National Health Service (NHS) in Wales (Chang et al., 2011).

The Welsh Government establishes the strategic framework and health and social care policies that NHS Wales and its partners follow. The NHS in Wales operates through seven Local Health Boards, three NHS Trusts, and two Special Health Authorities. The Local Health Boards are tasked with planning and ensuring the delivery of a range of services, including primary, community, and secondary care, as well as specialist services such as dentistry, optometry, pharmacy, and mental health. They work to improve health outcomes, promote well-being, and reduce health inequalities across their populations (NHS Confederation, 2021).

Public vs private

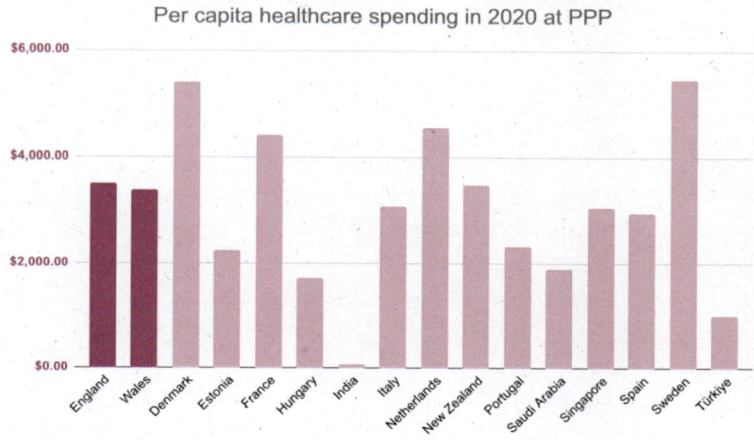

Figure 230. Source: The World Bank; *How well is the NHS in Wales performing?*

The national PHR

History

The Digital Services for Patients and the Public (DSPP) of NHS Wales creates Wales' version of England's NHS App. Welsh requirements included adding the Welsh language and different functionality. DSPP programme awarded the app development to Kainos, a software company that was also involved in the development of the NHS app in England.

Private beta with a thousand patients at 10 GP surgeries started in November 2022. At that stage, DSPP's priority was to ensure GPs understand the app's implications for their patients and take ownership of its integration into their practice.

Public beta testing started in April 2023. The app was available via the Apple and Google app stores. A web version is at app.nhs.wales in English and ap.gig.cymru in Welsh (Welsh Government, 2023).

Features

The GP practice must enable these for a patient to use: booking appointments, re-ordering repeat prescriptions, and seeing a summary of a patient's GP health record (NHS Wales App, 2024). The app also provides access to national information services, such as NHS 111 and organ donation services, where available.

- Appointments (the GP practice decides which appointment types are available):
    - Patients can request an appointment with their GP
    - Patients can cancel appointments with their GP through the app
- GP Prescriptions:
    - Patients can order a prescription
    - Patients can view their existing repeat prescriptions
    - Patients can view both current and past medicines

Depending on the health board or GP practice, patients may also be able to see:

- Medicines prescribed by their GP
- Any allergies or allergic reactions recorded by their GP
- Test results from their GP
- "My health timeline," which is a collection of all the patient's health records and events, searchable by date and record type

- "About me and my care," which is a form where patients can describe their healthcare needs, preferences, and plans
- The app also provides information on organ and blood donation services

Patients Know Best

Similar to the NHS App in England, the NHS Wales App integrates services and features developed by private companies. Notably, it relies on Patients Know Best (PKB) to provide patients with access to their test results, a library of health resources, symptom tracking, measurements, journal entries, care planning, and messaging. Additionally, screens include a direct link to PKB, allowing users to access all other PKB features from within the app. While the core functionality of the NHS Wales App enables patients to access their GP records, the integration with PKB allows them also to see data from other healthcare providers, including hospitals in Wales and providers in the rest of the UK.

This integration is still in progress and is currently available only in regions choosing PKB as the PHR provider. In these regions, patients can access parts of their PKB record within the NHS Wales App and use the NHS login's encrypted single sign-on for secure access.

Challenges and areas for improvement

The budget allocated by the Welsh government for the development of the NHS Wales App is smaller than that for the NHS App in England. As a result, there will be fewer features, and development will be slower.

The government's special health authority, Digital Health and Care Wales (DHCW), has locked down both the use of NHS login and access to the NHS Wales App. Agreements will be between Health

Boards and DHCW on behalf of apps or private sector providers rather than those providers getting single approval for use across Wales.

Therefore, the integration rollout will be slowed, which will lead to less private-sector collaboration. While the NHS Wales App should function as a single entry point for digital health and care services for all patients, this will result in unequal access across health boards during these slow rollouts (PKB research, 2024).

Published outcomes - statistics

At the beginning of December 2023, the NHS Wales App had (Digital Services for Patients and Public, 2023):

- 202 GP practices onboarded (52% of all practices in Wales), with a plan to onboard the remaining 48% within March 2024
- Over 50,000 app downloads by patients via App Store or Google Play Store
- 3,169 appointments have been booked through the app
- 15,855 repeat prescriptions have been ordered
- 48,519 GP health records have been viewed

Screenshots

Core NHS Wales App

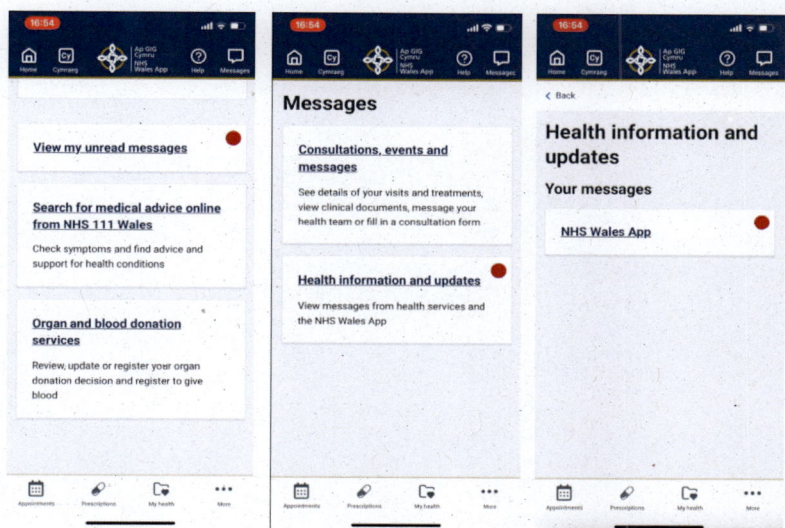

Figure 231. Patients can view their messages, search for medical advice through NHS 111 Wales, and review, update, or register their organ donation decisions. They also have the option to register as blood donors.

Figure 232. On the messages page, patients can access consultations, events, and messages, a service provided by Patients Know Best (PKB), as shown in the previous screenshots. Additionally, they can view health information and updates.

Figure 233. In the Health Information and Updates section, patients can see messages from the NHS Wales app.

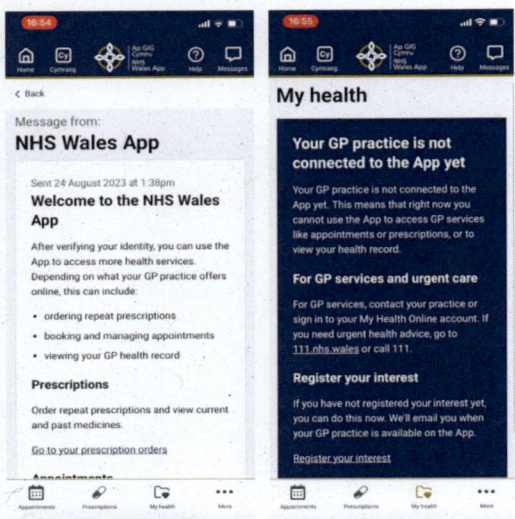

Figure 234. NHS Wales App shows a welcome message for patients.

Figure 235. Within 'My Health,' patients can determine whether their GP practice is connected to the App. If their practice is connected, they will have access to view appointments, prescriptions, and their health data.

Patients Know Best within the NHS Wales App

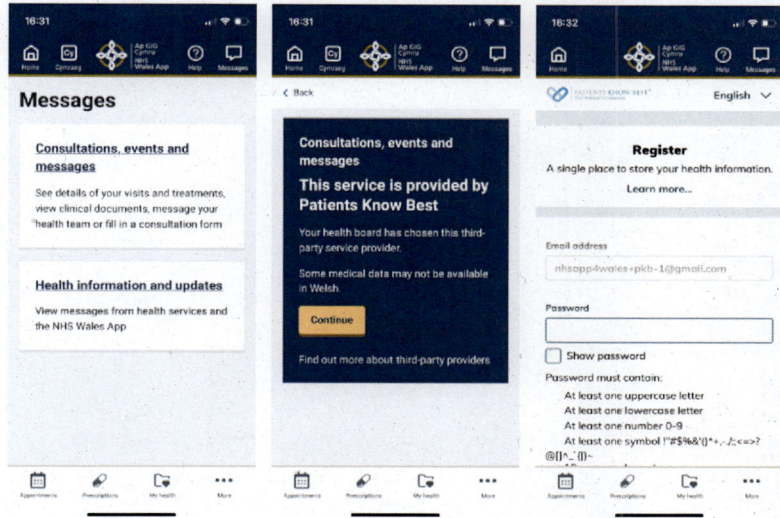

Figure 236. On the Messages Page, patients have two options for managing their communications. They can either click to view more details about their visits, treatments, and clinical documents, as well as send messages to their healthcare professionals, or they can select the option to view messages received from health services and the NHS Wales App.

Figure 237. Upon clicking on 'Consultations, Events, and Messages,' patients are notified that this service is provided by the company Patients Know Best (PKB).

Figure 238. When opening messages for the first time, patients are required to register with Patients Know Best (PKB).

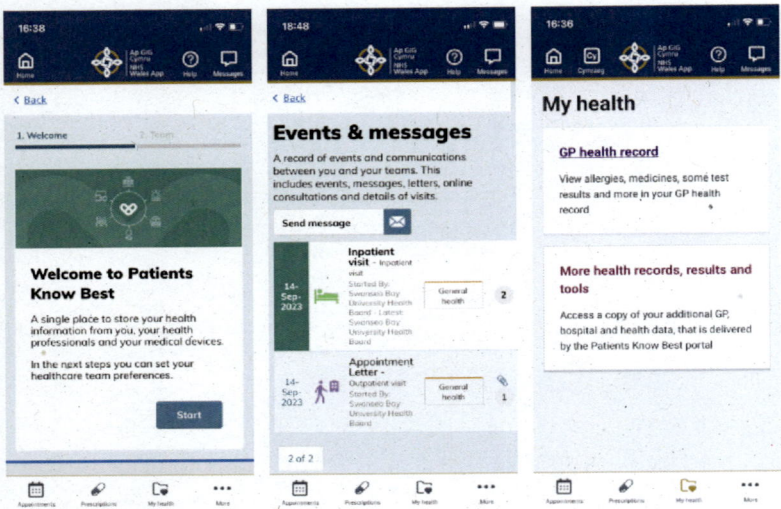

Figure 239. Once registered, patients can review their sharing settings and begin utilising all the services available through the NHS Wales app, as provided by Patients Know Best (PKB).

Figure 240. Once registered, patients are directed to the specific area of Patients Know Best (PKB) they selected from the NHS App, in this instance, the Events & Messages section. Here, they can view and send messages to their healthcare professionals, as well as access their letters.

Figure 241. In the 'My Health' menu, patients can click to access their GP health record or explore additional options under 'More health records, results, and tools.'

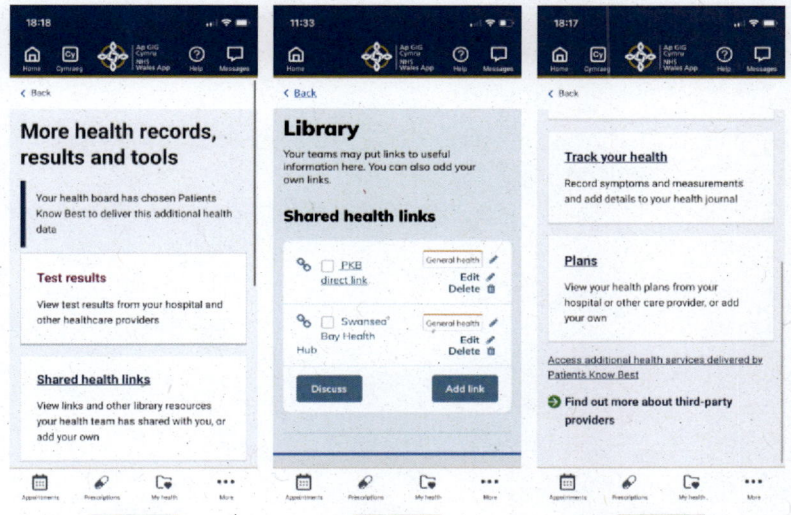

Figure 242. Upon clicking on 'More health records, results, and tools,' patients can select to view their test results or access a library of resources provided by their health team.

Figure 243. When clicking on 'Shared health links,' patients are presented with a library of links and files added by their healthcare professionals, as well as the option to add their own.

Figure 244. Patients have the option to click on 'Track your health' to record their symptoms, measurements, and journal entries. They can also select 'Plans' to view their health management plans.

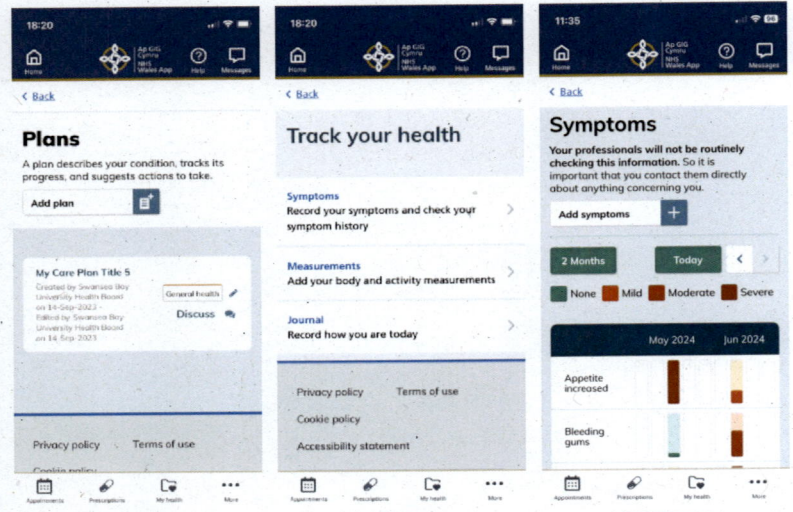

Figure 245. 'Plans' can outline the patient's condition, track their progress, and suggest actionable steps for management. Both healthcare professionals and patients can contribute to these plans.

Figure 246. The menu within 'Track your health' features options for 'symptoms,' 'measurements,' and 'journal,' allowing patients to monitor and document their health.

Figure 247. On the 'Symptoms' page, patients can input their symptoms along with an indication of their intensity.

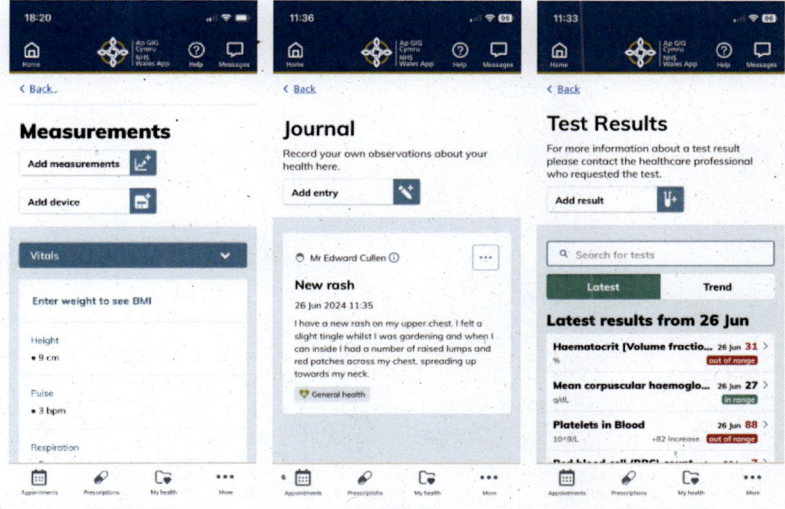

Figure 248. On the 'Measurements' page, patients have the option to manually enter their measurements or connect a device to track and record their data automatically.

Figure 249. In the 'Journal' page, patients can create new journal entries by typing in a free text box, allowing them to express their thoughts and observations about their health.

Figure 250. In the 'Test Results' page, patients can view results from past tests or manually add new ones. The results are displayed as a list and in graphs, enabling patients to track trends.

Bibliography

- Chang, J., Peysakhovich, F., Wang, W. and Zhu, J., 2011. The UK health care system. The United Kingdom, 30, p.2019. Available at: http://assets.ce.columbia.edu/pdf/actu/actu-uk.pdf (accessed: 2 August 2024).

- Cochrane, A. L. (1972). Effectiveness and Efficiency: Random Reflections on Health Services. London: Nuffield Provincial Hospitals Trust. Available at: https://www.nuffieldtrust.org.uk/sites/default/files/2017-01/effectiveness-and-efficiency-web-final.pdf (accessed: 2 November 2024).

- Digital Services for Patients and Public (2023) DSPP – Cynnydd ar App GIG Cymru // DSPP Webinar - Progress on the NHS Wales App. Available at: https://www.youtube.com/watch?v=56ZHsyROVv8 (accessed: 8 December 2023).

- Evenstad, L. (30 Mar 2023). Wales is building a dragon of an NHS app. Computerweekly. Available at: https://www.computerweekly.com/news/365534184/The-Welsh-are-building-a-dragon-of-an-NHS-app (accessed: 18 December 2023).

- NHS Wales App (2024) NHS Wales App: Help and support. Available at: https://apphelp.nhs.wales/ (accessed: 19 November 2024).

- NHS Confederation, 2021. About the NHS in Wales. (online) 12 May. Available at: https://www.nhsconfed.org/articles/about-nhs-wales (accessed: 2 August 2024).

- Welsh Government. (17 April 2023). Cabinet Statement: Written Statement - The new NHS Wales App, by Eluned Morgan MS, Minister for Health and Social Services. Available at: https://www.gov.wales/written-statement-new-nhs-wales-app (accessed: 18 December 2023).

AUTHORS

Federica Andreoni

Federica graduated with a Bachelor's degree in Business and Economics from the University of Bologna in 2019. In 2021, she completed a Master's degree in Innovation Management at the University of Trento and Sant'Anna in Pisa.

Currently, Federica is a Project Manager and manages the Patients Know Best Education Programme, the non-profit arm of the company.

Federica is also leading this research, focusing on the analysis of national PHRs from multiple countries.

Mohammad Al-Ubaydli

Mohammad is the co-founder of Patients Know Best and has over 27 years of experience in medical software. He trained as a physician at the University of Cambridge, worked as a staff scientist at the US National Institutes of Health, and ran the hospital chief information officer consulting practice for US hospitals at the Advisory Board Company.

Dr. Al-Ubaydli wrote 7 books about the use of IT in health care, including 'Personal Health Records: a Guide for Clinicians'.